An Illustrated Pocketbook of Pediatric Infectious Diseases

An Illustrated Pocketbook of Pediatric Infectious Diseases

Russell W. Steele

Professor and Vice Chairman of Pediatrics
Chief, Louisiana State University Infectious Disease Division
The Regional Medical Center for Children
New Orleans, Louisiana, USA

The Parthenon Publishing Group
International Publishers in Medicine, Science & Technology

A CRC PRESS COMPANY

BOCA RATON   LONDON   NEW YORK   WASHINGTON, D.C.

Published in the USA by
The Parthenon Publishing Group
345 Park Avenue South, 10th Floor
New York, NY 10010, USA

Published in the UK and Europe by
The Parthenon Publishing Group Limited
23–25 Blades Court
Deodar Road
London SW15 2NU, UK

Library of Congress Cataloging-in-Publication Data
Data available on application

British Library Cataloguing in Publication Data
Steele, Russell W. (Russell Wesley), 1942-
    An illustrated pocketbook of pediatric infectious diseases
    1. Communicable diseases in children
    I. Title
    618.9'29

ISBN 1-84214-140-6

Composition by The Parthenon Publishing Group
Printed and bound by T. G. Hostench S.A., Spain

Contents

Preface

In the care of pediatric patients, infectious diseases make up over half of diagnostic considerations. For this reason, the pediatrician or primary-care physician who is involved in the treatment of children must be particularly prepared with a basic understanding of infectious processes.

In many cases, knowledge of the disease must be applied in the clinical setting with a minimum of delay. These situations may be handled best by the physician who has access to a resource which contains a comprehensive collection of physical findings, radiographic illustrations and laboratory information pertinent to both the common as well as relatively uncommon infections. This Pocketbook provides the clinician with just such a resource, aided by the use of high-quality color photographs collected by the author and colleagues over many years of clinical practice.

This book contains information on over 150 carefully selected diseases with concomitant illustrations. Each topic is presented with concise yet complete diagnostic information, with an emphasis on the practical aspects of management. Recent data on newly emerging infectious diseases are also highlighted.

Included among the ten sections are infectious disease emergencies, congenital and perinatal infections, and presentations unique to the immunocompromised host. As an aid to the reader who is using the book to help in the diagnosis of specific patients with exanthematous diseases, additional sections are divided according to the characteristics of the rash.

This book will be an important educational and reference resource for medical students, primary-care physicians and residents who manage care for children. Furthermore, as all of these infectious diseases have been and will continue to be frequently encountered in medical practice, the information contained in this volume is unlikely to ever become out of date.

A Review of Pediatric Infectious Diseases

Congenital and perinatal infections

Serious infections are more common during the neonatal period than at any other time in life; this is largely a consequence of immature host defense mechanisms. During the first 28 days of life, the incidence of sepsis is reported to be as high as 8 cases per 1000 live births, with 20–25% of these having associated meningitis. Despite medical advances, mortality due to such infections remains at approximately 25%.

Neonatal sepsis can be divided into early-onset and late-onset disease. Late-onset sepsis typically affects previously healthy infants who have been discharged from the hospital. Early clinical manifestations of neonatal sepsis are frequently non-specific and subtle, and often show overlap with symptoms of non-infectious diseases. Well-defined perinatal factors identify which infants are at greatest risk for infection; for example, prematurity markedly increases risk.

Laboratory studies may be helpful during initial clinical evaluations, especially white blood cell (WBC) count and differential. An absolute neutrophil count < 1800/mm^3 or an immature neutrophil-to-total neutrophil ratio of > 0.15 during the first 24 h of life is strongly suggestive of infection. Leukocytosis, defined as a WBC count of > 25 000/mm^3, may also be the result of infection, but is more often associated with non-infectious causes.

Other hematological findings in neonatal infection include thrombobocytopenia, WBC vacuolization and toxic granulations. Rapid antigen detection tests, such as latex particle agglutination or countercurrent immunoelectrophoresis, offer supportive evidence for specific bacterial etiologies, but false-positive results have limited their usefulness. Numerous other adjunctive tests, including C-reactive protein and erythrocyte sedimentation rate (ESR) tests, have been used to screen for sepsis, but none have been widely accepted.

Cultures of blood and cerebrospinal fluid (CSF) should be obtained from all neonates with suspected sepsis, although clinical judgment should be exercised to determine the safety of lumbar puncture in infants at risk for respiratory compromise or preterm infants at risk from intraventricular hemorrhage. Tracheal aspirate cultures, when available, are useful in infants with respiratory symptoms, although endotracheal tube colonization is inevitable with prolonged intubation. Urine culture is of low yield in the evaluation of early-onset infection, but is useful in late-onset infection. Urine for culture should be obtained by suprapubic aspiration of the bladder if possible. Gastric aspirate and skin cultures may reflect bacterial colonization at birth, but do not always correlate with systemic infection. Chest radiography is indicated in infants with respiratory distress as a screen for both pneumonia and non-infectious causes.

Normal values for CSF in neonates differ from those in older infants. Cerebrospinal fluid WBC counts as high as $30/mm^3$, protein values of 170 mg/dl and glucose values as low as 24 mg/dl are normal during the neonatal period.

Congenital infections with non-bacterial pathogens also result in significant morbidity and mortality. TORCH is the acronym for what were once the more common pathogens involved in congenital infections: *Toxoplasma* species, rubella virus, cytomegalovirus (CMV), and herpes simplex virus.

Clinical manifestations of intrauterine infections are variable and there is considerable overlap among the different pathogens. Findings that should arouse suspicion for congenital disease include intrauterine growth retardation, microcephaly, hepatosplenomegaly, anemia and thrombocytopenia. It should be noted, however, that most cases of intrauterine growth retardation and microcephaly are not caused by infection.

Infectious disease emergencies

Some infectious disease presentations should be diagnosed and treated rapidly to prevent mortality and to provide the optimal prognosis. In many cases, therapy must be instituted before diagnosis can be confirmed. These are true emergencies and, fortunately, only a few such entities are commonly encountered in pediatric patients.

Sepsis and meningitis are the two most commonly seen emergencies. In most cases, only two laboratory specimens need to be obtained before treatment is begun. In other instances, only supportive therapy is warranted, either because specific treatment is not yet available or because eradication of the invading pathogen is not necessary. Such entities include viral encephalitis (other than herpes simplex virus or varicella-zoster virus), viral myocarditis, Reye syndrome, Guillain–Barré syndrome, infant botulism, and rabies.

The clinician's assessment of toxicity remains the most sensitive test for determining which children have early, but potentially severe, bacterial infections. Such assessment has been carefully defined and quantitated using criteria referred to as the eight-category Yale Observation Scale:

(1) Feeding history;

(2) Reaction to the environment;

(3) Irritability;

(4) Consolability;

(5) Absence of social smile;

(6) Quality of the cry;

(7) Color;

(8) Hydration.

A judgment that a child fulfills criteria for toxicity has an impact on decisions for the diagnostic work-up, such as cultures, measurement of, for example, acute-phase reactants, hospitalization and empirical antimicrobial therapy.

Streptococcus pneumoniae and *Neisseria meningitidis* are now the two bacterial organisms causing most cases of bacteremia which progress to shock with multi-organ failure or produce focal infection, such as meningitis, pneumonia, and purulent pericarditis. Other pathogens which have emerged as common etiologies of severe infection are group A beta-hemolytic streptococci and *Staphylococcus aureus*, half of which are resistant to methicillin.

Many of the bacterial infections included in the following illustrated section will progress to septic shock if not treated early and aggressively. Selection of empirical antibiotic therapy depends on the clinical setting, early clues for etiological diagnosis and on a thorough knowledge of microbial susceptibility patterns.

Most infectious disease emergencies should be managed in a well-equipped intensive care unit, at least during the acute phase. By definition, progression of disease may require endotracheal intubation or other specialized support procedures. For this reason, transport to referral medical centers should be considered.

Maculopapular exanthematous diseases

The rashes of the exanthematous diseases of childhood can be broadly separated into those which are primarily erythematous maculopapular and those which are papulovesicular. These classifications represent the starting point used by clinicians in formulating a differential diagnosis during initial examination and management. Additional data for diagnosis are the prodrome, other diagnostic signs and laboratory tests.

The following are the most common and most often misdiagnosed diseases associated with maculopapular rashes:

Drug eruptions   Enteroviral infections

Epstein–Barr virus infections   Erythema infectiosum

Erythema multiforme minor	Kawasaki disease
Measles	Roseola
Staphylococcal scaled skin syndrome	Scarlet fever
	Rubella

Macular rashes that mimic measles (morbilli) are often referred to as morbilliform eruptions. Macules are otherwise defined as color changes of the skin that are flat (not palpable), whereas papules are raised with distinct borders measuring 1 cm or less. Many exanthems exhibit a combination of macules and papules, and are thus referred to as maculopapular eruptions.

Viruses induce skin rashes either by direct invasion of the skin, where they replicate within keratinocytes (epidermotropic), or by indirectly producing skin reactivity by poorly defined mechanisms. Lesions are usually generalized. However, the majority have a photodistribution, as exposure to the sun enhances their intensity.

Maculopapular eruptions are the most common form of viral-induced exanthems and therefore constitute the most frequent differential diagnosis. Many maculopapular eruptions are of non-infectious etiology, most commonly induced by drugs. Because of their frequent use, antibiotics are often incriminated. Reactive erythema due to trauma or sensitivity to sunlight may also mimic viral exanthems.

Papulovesicular exanthematous diseases

Papules and vesicles are sharply circumscribed elevated lesions < 1 cm in diameter. Vesicles contain non-purulent fluid. Often, these lesions evolve from papules to vesicles that rupture to produce ulcerated craters, scales, or crusts. Secondary colonization with common skin flora, particularly *S. aureus* and group A streptococci, may produce impetigo, cellulitis or subcutaneous abscesses.

Papulovesicular eruptions often present with many stages of development and a combination of secondary features. Non-infectious etiologies are numerous. Examples of lesions that are papular, but non-vesicular, are nevi and lichen planus. The most common entities that vesiculate include dyshydrosis and contact dermatitis. Many viral and bacterial pathogens produce papular and/or vesicular exanthems. One of these, smallpox or variola, was successfully eradicated world-wide but is now of concern because of its potential for use in a bioterrorist attack. The most common and often misdiagnosed diseases characterized by papulovesicular eruptions are:

Coxsackie virus infections	Eczema herpeticum
Gianotti–Crosti syndrome	Herpetic whitlow
Impetigo	Molluscum contagiosum
Papular urticaria	Varicella-zoster

Clinical features that help to differentiate infections should be particularly noted. These include the distribution of the rash, associated enanthems, presence of fever, or other constitutional symptoms and unique associated findings.

Enanthems

Examination of the oral cavity not only provides information on patients whose primary complaint relates to the mouth and throat, but may also yield important diagnostic clues to systemic disease. The state of hydration may be assessed by the amount of moisture on mucous membranes; the pallor of anemia may be noted, and cyanosis of the lips is evidence of congenital heart disease. Malodorous breath is associated with tissue breakdown from infection, particularly anaerobes (e.g. Vincent's angina), but may also provide the first indication of liver disease or diabetes mellitus.

Lesions in the oral cavity may be structural defects, inflammatory, neoplastic or post-traumatic as well as of infectious etiology. In addition, there are some non-infectious etiologies that have appearances similar to enanthems (see later).

One of the most common structural abnormalities is the mucocele which are lesions at the site of minor salivary glands. Epstein pearls are white nodular cystic structures located along the alveolar ridge in young infants, and dermoid cysts may appear along the anterior floor of the mouth. A torus palatinus is a bony defect of the hard palate seen in 20% of adolescents, and a fibrosing mucocele is a similar developmental abnormality of the mucous membrane covering the palate.

The most common inflammatory disorder is erythema multiforme of the mouth, often associated with a skin rash and conjunctivitis. The severe form is called Stevens–Johnson syndrome. Other common inflammatory lesions include gingival hyperplasia and lichen planus.

Most important among the differentials are malignant neoplasms, but these are generally larger masses. Unlike oral tumors in adults, the lesions in children are usually sarcomas, with rhabdomyosarcoma predominating. With tissue breakdown, these may be confused with abscesses, cellulitis, or other infectious lesions.

Trauma to the oral mucosa and injuries from sharp objects such as pencils or popsicle sticks are most likely to imitate enanthems associated with infectious diseases. A careful history for trauma should thus be obtained if lesions are not completely characteristic of other etiologies.

Sexually transmitted diseases

Sexually transmitted diseases (STDs) can be broadly divided into those characterized by genital ulcers with or without inguinal adenopathy, infections of epithelial surfaces, and specific well-defined syndromes. Genital ulcers are most commonly associated with herpes simplex, syphilis or, less commonly, chancroid, and may be differentiated by the presence or absence of pain. Syphilis is usually painless, whereas herpes and chancroid are painful.

Depending on the specific findings and other features such as adenopathy (syphilis, lymphogranuloma venereum (LGV) and chancroid), evaluation of genital ulcers should include the following: dark-field examination or direct immunofluorescence tests for *Treponema pallidum*; serological tests for syphilis; culture or fluorescence stains for herpes simplex virus (HSV); and culture for *Haemophilus ducreyi*.

The appearance of the skin lesions is often diagnostic. Genital warts (papillomavirus), ecchymoses of the arthritis–dermatitis syndrome (*N. gonorrhoeae*) and the multiple painful ulcers of HSV are readily recognizable.

STDs may also be classified according to their specific pathogens, but this is less practical than an etiological diagnosis on the basis of clinical presentations. An example is urethritis, which may be the result of bacteria, viruses or even protozoa.

The classical STD triad of syphilis, gonorrhea and chancroid now accounts for only a fraction of the currently recognized pathogens. Indeed, they have been largely replaced by Papillomavirus, *Chlamydia trachomatis*, and hepatitis B as major diseases.

With the increasing prevalence of STDs, physicians have emphasized methods of prevention, particularly among adolescents, and have become more aware of the variable presentations, the potential seriousness of the sequelae for children born to infected mothers, and the implications of the diagnosis of an acquired STD in a prepubescent child in terms of child abuse.

Because multiple STDs frequently coexist in the same patient, the detection of one disease requires examination for others, regardless of the presenting symptoms. Careful physical examination, including the oropharynx, rectum, genitalia and skin, should be performed. Laboratory studies include urinalysis, selected serological tests based on clinical findings, Gram stains of cervical and urethral discharge, wet mounts of vaginal secretions, diagnostic tests for *C. trachomatis* on cervical (vaginal in prepubertal girls) or urethral specimens, and cultures of the oropharynx, rectum and cervix or penile urethra for *N. gonorrhoeae*. The detection of HIV infection often alters the management of STDs, particularly syphilis, which would then require higher dosages of penicillin and a longer duration of therapy.

It is frequently forgotten that infection in a neonate or young infant with a pathogen that is transmitted through sexual contact warrants evaluation and treatment of the mother as well as her sexual contacts. Examples include gonococcal ophthalmia, chlamydial conjunctivitis and pneumonia, congenital syphilis and HIV. Mothers with these infections are frequently asymptomatic.

STDs in children may have been acquired by sexual contact. Studies suggest that approximately 20% of children and adolescents have been sexually abused by the age of 21 years. Sexual abuse is generally perpetrated by someone known to the child and frequently continues over a prolonged period. If the sexual abuse event occurred more that 72 h before evaluation, specimens should be collected for evaluation of the common STDs. If the abuse was more recent, then the appropriate forensic specimens should be collected. Antimicrobial treatments should be considered if:

(1)   The alleged perpetrator was known to be infected with an STD;

(2)   More than one assailant was involved;

(3)   The patient is unlikely to return for follow-up;

(4)   The patient or parents are anxious regarding the possibility of acquiring an STD.

When evaluating a child for possible sexual abuse, appropriate tests for gonorrhea, chlamydial infection, HIV and syphilis (as well as for other infections in selected circumstances) should be obtained. Evaluating physicians should identify those patients suspected of being victims of sexual abuse who thus warrant laboratory evaluation for an STD. Some experts advise culturing all children for *C. trachomatis* and *N. gonorrhoeae* as many abused children do not disclose the extent of their abuse, and infection with these agents may be asymptomatic.

Skin, soft tissue and lymph node infections

Infectious diseases that affect the skin and skin structures allow ready application of diagnostic skills, microscopic evaluation and culture of the offending pathogen. In addition, some diseases are associated with skin lesions as a result of toxin production, immune complex formation or delayed hypersensitivity reactions to antigens from responsible microbes.

Soft-tissue infections may be the result of direct inoculation of the skin, bacteremia and hematogenous spread from another site, lymphogenous proliferation of pathogens, or extension from contiguous disease. Microorganisms may produce abscesses, affect vascular structures causing visible changes or alter extravascular structures of the dermis.

Many factors need to be borne in mind when making early clinical diagnoses. Characteristics of the skin lesions are the first consideration. Vesicular, bullous, petechial, pustular, ulcerated or nodular lesions each suggest a specific etiology in a differential diagnosis. The location of the lesions separates many similar entities: chronic submandibular adenopathy is more indicative of atypical mycobacterial disease, whereas similar lymphatic involvement in the axillae is suggestive of cat-scratch disease.

When a specific etiology is strongly suspected on clinical grounds alone and the patient is asymptomatic or only mildly ill, an empirical course of therapy without further diagnostic testing is appropriate. This significantly reduces the cost of medical care. Most of the infections included in this book fall into this category. Laboratory confirmation may only be necessary to identify unusual antimicrobial susceptibility patterns or to separate a few possibilities within a differential diagnosis.

Infections specific to organ systems

Young children often develop infection with common colonizing bacteria because they lack antibody to these organisms and because their immune responses are decreased compared with those of adults. Important potential pathogens include *Streptococcus pneumoniae*, *H. influenzae*, *N. meningitidis*, *S. aureus* and group A β-hemolytic streptococci. These five groups predominate in children during the preschool years following infancy, and are responsible for bacteremia, sepsis and serious focal infections, such as cellulitis, pericarditis, osteomyelitis, pneumonia and meningitis.

With any febrile illness, it is important that the clinician look for clues that may differentiate the usual self-limited viral infections from bacterial disease of greater consequence. This is generally achieved by assessment of 'toxicity', as the child with early bacterial infection is more likely to manifest clinical changes indicative of infection of greater consequence:

(1) Feeding history;

(2) State of hydration;

(3) Reaction to the environment;

(4) Irritability;

(5) Consolability;

(6) Absence of a social smile;

(7) Quality of the cry;

(8) Color changes (such as pallor and cyanosis).

The sensitivity of this clinical assessment is approximately 75% for determining serious illness, which is higher than that of any laboratory test currently available.

The site of infection may not cause obvious focal signs and symptoms; examples are urinary tract infection, brain abscesses and osteomyelitis. Therefore, for any patient with a suspected bacterial illness, blood cultures should be obtained. However, even in cases with an obvious focus, blood cultures may be positive, whereas the local site may prove negative on culture.

Early antibiotic therapy for children with a high fever, but no identifiable focus of infection, remains highly controversial. Although some studies have shown benefit with early empirical therapy, the increasing antibiotic resistance of organisms such as S. *pneumoniae* to commonly used agents for treatment argues against their routine use in all children considered at risk for occult bacteremia. It would probably be best for the physician to individualize cases by examining all young children carefully for toxicity and for early signs of focal disease.

Other infectious diseases

Non-bacterial pathogens account for a significant percentage of infections in children. These are predominantly viruses, which comprise the etiology of most upper and lower respiratory tract infections, and most self-limited febrile illnesses.

Although fungal diseases constitute a small percentage of disease, they may be life-threatening, particularly if diagnosis is delayed. *Pneumocystis carinii*, now classified as a fungus, is the predominant cause of life-threatening pneumonia in children with HIV infection, and is usually treated with trimethoprim-sulfamethoxazole. Other mycoses are treated with amphotericin B, imadazoles (clotrimazole, miconazole and ketoconazole) or triazoles (fluconazole and itraconazole).

Rickettsiae are unique bacterial pathogens and are treated with tetracyclines or chloramphenicol. Antimicrobial therapy for these pathogens is therefore very different from that required for some bacterial pathogens, for which the cephalosporins or penicillins are usually employed. However, none of the rickettsiae are susceptible to these classes of antibiotics.

Parasitic diseases have virtually disappeared in the developed countries as a result of improved sanitary conditions. Malaria and intestinal nematodes are now encountered in patients who have traveled to tropical developing countries. Only pinworm (enterobiasis) and giardiasis are seen with any frequency in US pediatric practices, with occasional cases of ascariasis, amebiasis, strongyloidiasis, toxocariasis, hookworm and whipworm requiring management.

The immunocompromised host

Reduced host defense responses may be the result of congenital abnormalities (primary immunodeficiency) or may be secondary to certain disease processes, such as cancer and autoimmune disorders, wherein host responses are worsened by the immunosuppressive chemotherapy.

Initial clinical manifestations are often infections due to pathogens that are rarely seen in the immune-competent host or severe disease caused by relatively non-virulent microbial agents. The type of pathogen (viral, fungal, extracellular bacteria or intracellular bacteria) often suggests the compartment of immune function – cellular, humoral or phagocytic – that is most affected.

It is difficult to determine the incidence of primary immunodeficiency syndromes as many of the more severe forms may result in early infant death before diagnosis can be made. In one study, it was estimated that one in 50 deaths in children was a result of immune dysfunction.

In clinical practice, however, the more severe defects are only occasionally encountered by primary-care physicians. It is the more common deficiencies, such as transient hypogammaglobulinemia of infancy and selective IgA deficiency, that are familiar to most clinicians. Other syndromes more likely to be encountered include common variable hypogammaglobulinemia, chronic mucocutaneous candidiasis, cyclic neutropenia, Brunton's X-linked hypogamma-globulinemia, severe combined immune deficiency, Wiscott–Aldrich syndrome and complement deficiencies.

The importance of measuring immune competence is more greatly appreciated as defects in immunity become increasingly implicated in disease processes. More importantly, early recognition of immune deficiency is critical for successful treatment of patients, both in terms of managing the primary disease and anticipating secondary complications.

Initial presentations may be subtle. On retrospective reviewing of the clinical histories of patients with documented immunodeficiency, it becomes apparent that the first encounter with a physician is for treatment of an apparently trivial illness such as pneumonia, a focal bacterial infection, a prolonged viral illness, or perhaps simply oral thrush.

All physicians should, as part of patient management, consider etiology and ask why this particular patient should have developed this particular disease. If the reason for the predisposition is apparent (it is the patient's first encounter with influenza virus resulting in pneumonia), then a satisfactory answer is available. If an explanation is not apparent (the patient has *P. carinii* pneumonia), then the physician should consider a thorough screen of immune function in this patient.

Most of these deficiencies present during infancy or early childhood; the most notable exceptions are common variable hypogammaglobulinemia, cyclic neutropenia and complement deficiencies, all of which may not become clinically apparent until later in life.

Deficiencies of the later components of complement (C5–8) are not seen until adolescence or early adulthood, with the presentation of recurrent meningococcal and gonococcal disease.

Secondary suppression of immunological function with resultant increased susceptibility to infection may occur as a result of a number of primary diseases. Oncology patients and others receiving immunosuppressive therapy have been evaluated to stage their susceptibility to infectious diseases in a manner similar to staging the prognosis in cancer. These are the patients who later may come to demonstrate disseminated varicella-zoster, *P. carinii* pneumonia, disseminated herpes simplex or bacterial sepsis.

Antimicrobial prophylaxis and early treatment are important aspects in management of such patients. Some will also benefit from such immunotherapeutic approaches as intravenous immunoglobulin or granulocyte colony-stimulating factor. This circumstance is more common in adults than in children because of the higher incidence of malignancy and greater use of immunosuppressive chemotherapy for a variety of diseases. The acquired immunodeficiency syndrome (AIDS) is the most common predisposing immunodeficiency in children.

Over 2% of all hospitalized children demonstrate secondary defects in host resistance. Recognition and treatment of these host defense abnormalities have therefore become an important aspect of hospital practice. Secondary deficiency is, in fact, much more common than primary immunological disorder in infants and children, and can be adequately managed by primary-care physicians with consultative support.

Pediatric Infectious Diseases Illustrated

Congenital and perinatal infections

Conjunctivitis

The causes of conjunctivitis are largely age-dependent in neonates and young infants, and include sensitivity to topical chemicals and environmental allergens as well as viral and bacterial pathogens. The most common etiology during the first 3 days of life is the prophylactic application of silver nitrate (Figure 1) and, to a lesser extent, erythromycin or tetracycline; no treatment is necessary.

From 3 days to 3 weeks of life, *Neisseria gonorrhoeae* produces ophthalmia neonatorum, which is best confirmed by Gram staining (Figure 2) and culture of a conjunctival scraping. *Chlamydia*

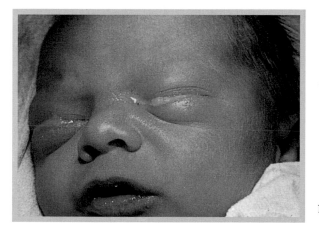

Figure 1

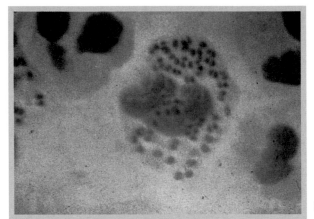

Figure 2

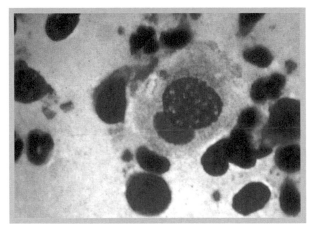

Figure 3

trachomatis produces conjunctivitis (inclusion blennorrhea) at 3–20 weeks of age. Identification can be made by Giemsa staining of a conjunctival scraping to reveal paranuclear elementary bodies within the epithelial cells (Figure 3). However, this method has only a 30% sensitivity compared with culture or direct fluorescent staining. Other causes of bacterial conjunctivitis after day 2 of life are *Staphylococcus aureus*, streptococci and coliforms.

Cytomegalovirus

Cytomegalovirus (CMV) may be vertically transmitted to the fetus during primary or recurrent maternal infection, but only 4% of infected infants are symptomatic at birth. These infants have a mortality rate of 25% and almost all survivors have long-term morbidity. Of the 96% of infected infants who are asymptomatic at birth, up to 15% will develop significant late neurological sequelae, with sensorineural hearing loss being the most common. Diagnosis is confirmed by recovery of CMV from the urine or a target organ.

An infant, who was small for gestational age, had congenital CMV infection and presented with the classical features of purpura, hepatosplenomegaly, microcephaly, severe anemia, thrombocytopenia and leukocytosis. Chest X-ray revealed interstitial infiltrates. CMV was cultured from the urine. Failure to thrive, respiratory distress, recurrent epistaxis and ascites persisted; death ensued at 9 weeks of age.

Other manifestations of congenital infection are jaundice (Figure 4), chorioretinitis and intracerebral, usually periventricular, calcifications. Another rare but specific radiological finding is intrahepatic calcifications.

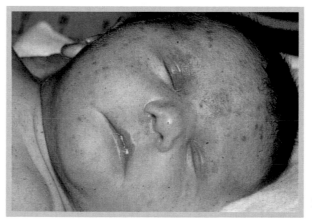

Figure 4

27

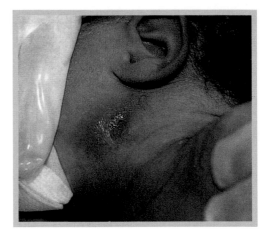

Figure 5

Group B streptococcal cellulitis–adenitis in infants

A unique presentation of infection due to group B streptococcus (GBS) in pediatric patients < 3 months of age (Figure 5) was originally termed 'facial submandibular cellulitis in young infants'. Illness begins with fever, irritability and decreased feeding, rapidly followed by swelling and erythema in the facial, submandibular or inguinal region. Local adenitis is a prominent feature and often provides a source of culture and identification of GBS.

Similar infection caused by *Staphylococcus aureus* rarely causes nodes to suppurate or to require surgical drainage. Two other contrasting features are that almost all patients with GBS disease are bacteremic, and the majority develop ipsilateral otitis media. The age of these pediatric patients (< 3 months old) should also differentiate them from those with other etiologies.

The mean age of onset is 5 weeks. There is a prevalence of serotype III strains, and recovery of the same organism from the maternal vaginal and/or rectal cultures is frequent, all of which serve to support cellulitis–adenitis as another manifestation of late-onset GBS disease transmitted by the mother. Management should therefore include a sepsis work-up with examination of the CSF, and careful evaluation of bones and joints to rule out other foci of infection.

Group B streptococci are the leading cause of early-onset sepsis in neonates and most commonly present as severe pneumonia during the first 48 h of life. Pulmonary infection may occasionally produce a diaphragmatic hernia. In a 10-day-old neonate, computed tomography (CT) of the chest confirmed protrusion of the liver through a defect in the right diaphragm and severe pneumonia at 2 h of life required intubation and antimicrobial therapy. Multiple blood cultures were positive for GBS. The hernia was not present prior to day 10 of life.

Herpes simplex viruses

Herpes simplex viruses (HSV) types 1 (15%) and 2 (85%) cause maternal herpes genitalis and may result in perinatal infection. Neonatal disease presents during the first 42 days of life as a rapidly evolving disease with clinical symptoms similar to those of bacterial sepsis. Most infected infants are born to mothers who are asymptomatic, but who shed the virus from a reactivated genital infection at the time of delivery.

Neonatal disease may be categorized into three classifications: localized infection of the skin (Figure 6), eyes or mouth; central nervous system (CNS) infection with or without skin, eye or mouth involvement; and disseminated infection. Mortality is highest for

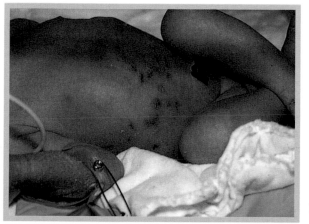

Figure 6

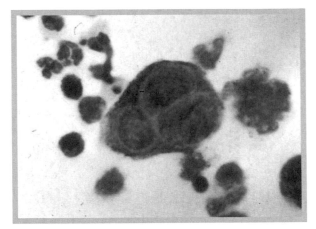

Figure 7

infants with disseminated disease and morbidity is high for infants with disseminated or CNS infection.

Diagnosis can be confirmed by culture of the virus from skin vesicles, mucosal lesions, blood or CSF. Skin lesions may be subtle; one neonate had a single vesicle behind the ear. Cytological examination with fluorescence, or a Tzanck preparation using Wright or Giemsa staining of the lesion scrapings, may also be helpful in diagnosis by identifying multinucleated giant cells (Figure 7).

An infant had encephalitis diagnosed at age 6 days. HSV type 2 was recovered from vesicles in the axilla. The infant developed profound mental retardation and death occurred 3 months later. No anti-microbial therapy was given.

Another presentation is bronchopneumonia, as in a severely ill neonate who had no skin manifestations or other organ involvement. Herpes may occasionally manifest as a true congenital infection following infection *in utero* during the first or second trimester of pregnancy, and cause growth retardation and deep dermal scars (Figure 8).

Neonatal tetanus

The neonate in Figure 9 developed opisthotonus 4 days after delivery. His umbilical cord had been cut by a midwife using an unsterilized

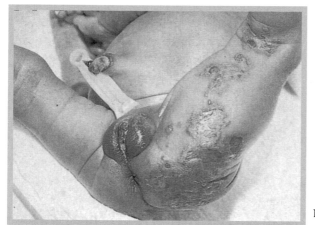

Figure 8

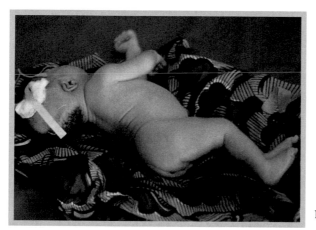

Figure 9

instrument and his mother had never received tetanus immunization. The causative organism is *Clostridium tetani*, present in the environment primarily in the form of spores, and lack of immunization, i.e. anti-tetanus antibody, is the greatest risk factor. Once introduced into a wound, however, the spores convert to the vegetative form, producing the potent toxin tetanospasmin. This affects the CNS, causing a variety of neurological and systemic manifestations, including seizures, and spasm of laryngeal and respiratory musculature, with airway obstruction, fever, tachycardia, hypertension, cardiac arrhythmias, and urinary retention.

The most commonly affected cranial nerves are III, IV, VII, IX and XI. The incubation period is 3 days to 3 weeks. Neonates usually present during the first week of life with difficulty in sucking, dysphagia, excessive crying, spasms and opisthotonus.

Mortality for neonatal tetanus is 80–90%. The condition is common in countries where women do not receive tetanus immunization, and accounts for an estimated 600 000 deaths per year. Recovery from tetanus does not confer immunity, so active immunization still needs to be offered.

Omphalitis

This is an infection of the umbilical stump, usually caused by *Staphylococcus aureus*, group A β-hemolytic or group B streptococci, or Gram-negative enteric bacilli, and may extend into the umbilical and portal veins to produce bacteremia and sepsis. Omphalitis is a true medical emergency. Infection of the umbilical cord without extension (funisitis) presents at birth in association with chorioamnionitis, whereas omphalitis tends to develop after 3–10 days.

Rubella

Transplacentally acquired during the course of primary maternal disease, rubella virus infection during fetal development may result in growth retardation, heart defects, hepatosplenomegaly, thrombo-cytopenia, cataracts, glaucoma and deafness. The incidence and severity of malformations are increased if infection occurs early in gestation.

Diagnosis can be made by testing for IgM antibody to rubella. Treatment is supportive and infected infants require isolation as virus excretion may be prolonged.

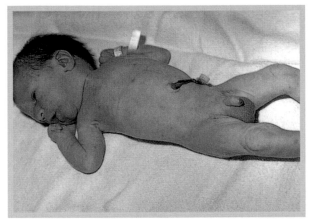

Figure 10

One such infant (Figure 10) had a low birth weight (2045 g at term), microcephaly, hepatosplenomegaly, lymphadenopathy, thrombocytopenia, peripheral pulmonic stenosis, cataracts and 'blueberry muffin' skin lesions (dermal erythropoiesis) on the face, chest, abdomen and legs.

Another child had congenital rubella with similar involvement, but with a patent ductus arteriosus, and 'blueberry muffin' skin lesions on the buttocks and leg. Figure 11 is an X-ray of the lower extremities of this infant and shows 'celery stalking' of the metaphyseal areas of the long bones, characteristic of congenital rubella. These linear radiolucencies disappear after 2–3 months.

Cataracts (Figure 12) and glaucoma (Figure 13), presenting at birth with large cloudy corneas, are suggestive of congenital rubella, although other congenital infections may also cause eye abnormalities.

Scalp abscess

Fetal monitoring with internal scalp electrodes, scalp blood sampling and trauma may result in a break in the skin with subsequent abscess formation. Group B streptococci, *Salmonella* species, *Escherichia coli* and *S. aureus* are the pathogens most frequently recovered from

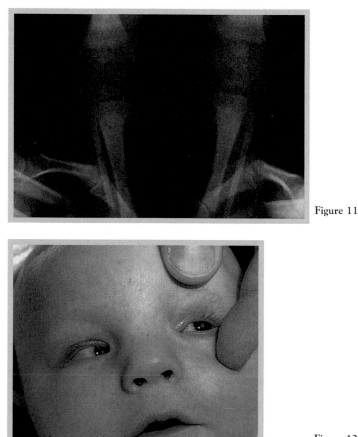

Figure 11

Figure 12

abscesses and/or blood. HSV or *N. gonorrhoeae* may cause infection when the mother is infected by these organisms.

A full-term infant with trisomy 21 (Down syndrome) had a cephalohemotoma measuring 3 x 4 cm at birth. Delivery by low forceps was uncomplicated. Fever, lethargy, anorexia and a rapidly enlarging scalp abscess were noted on day 11 of life. A complete blood count revealed 20 000 WBC/mm^3, with a marked shift to the left;

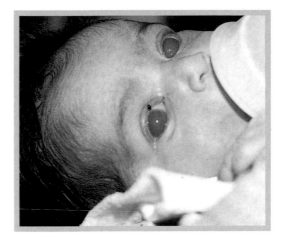

Figure 13

hemoglobin decreased from 19 g/dl to 14 g/dl, and the platelet count was 10 000/mm³. Moderate hepatosplenomegaly persisted for 4 weeks. Incision and drainage produced 200 ml of purulent material with a hydrogen sulfide odor. Cultures of blood and abscess material produced a heavy growth of *E. coli*. Recovery was rapid and examination at age 2 months was normal.

Syphilis

Congenital syphilis has shown a resurgence in recent years that has been indirectly associated with the illicit-drug epidemic. Transplacental passage of this spirochete may result in fetal wastage, non-immune hydrops or postnatal manifestations such as snuffles (Figure 14), rash, hepatitis and osteochondritis/periostitis (Figure 15). If syphilitic infection is left untreated, late manifestations will include neurosyphilis, deafness, and dental and bone abnormalities.

Infants infected with syphilis at birth are usually asymptomatic. Evaluation of maternal serology and therapy is therefore essential to identify them and prevent subsequent complications. All suspect infants should be assessed for congenital syphilis, initially with a non-treponemal serological test (e.g. Venereal Disease Research

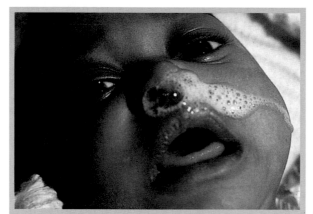

Figure 14

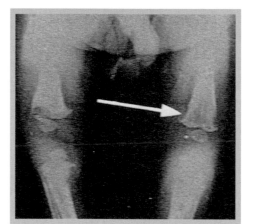

Figure 15

Laboratory (VDRL) test, automated reagin test (ART) or rapid plasma reagin (RPR) test) with positive responses confirmed using a specific treponemal test (e.g. the microhemagglutination assay (MHA-TP) or fluorescent treponemal antibody absorption (FTA-ABS) test). High-risk patients should only be tested with specific treponemal methodology.

Non-treponemal tests provide quantitative titers that correlate with disease activity, whereas treponemal tests provide confirmation of positive non-treponemal results and remain reactive for life, despite therapy. Evaluation of infants at risk should include physical examination, non-treponemal screening assay, MHA-TP or FTA-ABS, lumbar puncture, long bone and chest X-rays. CSF findings suggestive of neurosyphilis include leukocytosis, elevated protein or a positive VDRL test.

Condyloma lata are flat, moist lesions on the mucous membranes, and mucocutaneous areas of the male and female genitalia and perianal area. These lesions are indicative of secondary syphilis.

Dark-field examination of the condylomata and nasal secretions in the child with congenital syphilis and snuffles shown in Figure 14 showed them to be teeming with highly infectious spirochetes.

TORCH infections

Congenital infections with bacterial and non-bacterial pathogens may result in significant morbidity and mortality. TORCH (*Toxoplasma* species, rubella virus, CMV and NSV) has become less useful with the changing incidence of common pathogens involved in congenital infections.

CMV, the most commonly implicated agent in congenital infection, is estimated to infect 1–2% of all newborns in the USA. The increased prevalence of STDs such as syphilis and HIV has resulted in increasing numbers of newborns infected with these pathogens. At the same time, screening and immunization have all but eliminated rubella as a cause of congenital infection.

Clinical manifestations of congenital infection are variable and there is considerable overlap among potential pathogens. The classical triad is jaundice, hepatosplenomegaly and petechial rash (Figure 16). Neonates who are small for gestational age (SGA) also warrant examination for congenital infection, particularly when associated with microcephal (as in the infant with congenital rubella in Figure 10).

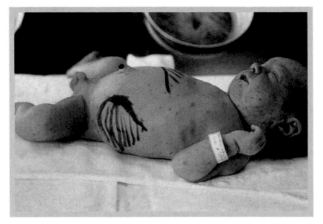

Figure 16

Toxoplasmosis

Toxoplasma gondii infection in the newborn occurs in approximately 1/1000 deliveries in the USA, as a result of transplacental transmission during maternal primary infection. Most infected infants are asymptomatic in infancy. Chorioretinitis occurs in > 80% of symptomatic infants. Other early clinical manifestations include hepatosplenomegaly, lymphadenopathy, a maculopapular or petechial rash and jaundice.

The child shown in Figure 17 developed hydrocephalus, successfully controlled by a ventriculo-peritoneal shunt at age 4 weeks. Skull X-rays were normal, but Gram staining of the CSF sediment revealed *Toxoplasma* organisms. Concentrations of IgM antibody specific for *T. gondii* were elevated. CT of the head at 4 months of age (Figure 18) showed marked dilatation of the ventricles, with multiple calcifications and scattered hypodense areas of cerebritis. Slow motor development persisted, with the infant's demise at age 14 months, in spite of treatment with sulfadiazine and pyrimethamine.

Varicella-zoster

Infection *in utero* from primary maternal varicella (chickenpox) during the first 20 weeks of pregnancy has occasionally been reported

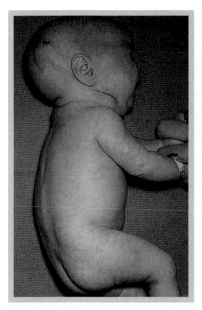

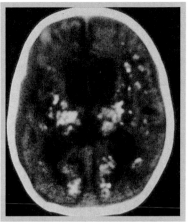

Figure 18

Figure 17

to result in an embryopathy characterized by cicatrices and limb paralysis with atrophy. Central nervous system and eye manifestations are also described. The most critical period is 9–16 weeks of gestation. Data are not available to define the magnitude of risk, but it appears to be less than 10%.

Chickenpox in a mother, beginning 5 days before to 2 days after delivery, may result in severe infection in the neonate at or shortly after birth (Figure 19). Such newborns should receive varicella-zoster immune globulin as soon as possible after delivery.

When a mother has chickenpox during pregnancy, apparently unaffected neonates exposed to the virus later in life may present with unusual manifestations of the disease, as in Figure 20, where the infant presented with vesicular lesions confined to the lower right extremity.

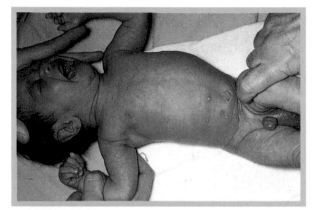

Figure 19

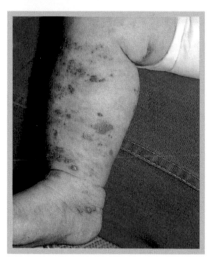

Figure 20

Infectious disease emergencies

Infant botulism

Disease in infants caused by *Clostridium botulinum* was first reported in 1976 and is now the most common form of botulism in the USA. The peak age of incidence is 6–8 weeks and nearly all reported cases have occurred in infants aged from 4 to 28 weeks.

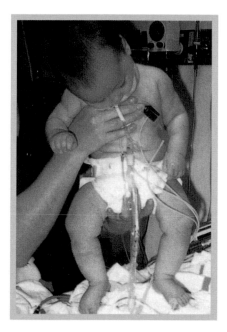

Figure 21

Disease begins with constipation, followed by poor feeding, and is frequently complicated by aspiration pneumonia and flaccid paralysis of the facial muscles. This is best appreciated when the infant is held erect, as this accentuates ptosis and causes the facial features to sag with gravity. There may also be oculomotor paralysis, with fixed stare and widely dilated pupils followed by flaccid paralysis of the trunk and limbs (Figure 21).

Electromyography characteristically shows brief, small abundant motor unit potentials (BSAP), which are considered pathognomonic (Figure 22). The definitive diagnosis is made by demonstration of C. *botulinum* toxin in the stool. C. *botulinum* organisms may be recovered from the stool using special egg yolk medium, wherein colonies exhibit a characteristic opalescent sheen. Staining of these colonies reveals large Gram-positive bacilli with bulging subterminal spores, producing a 'drumstick' appearance.

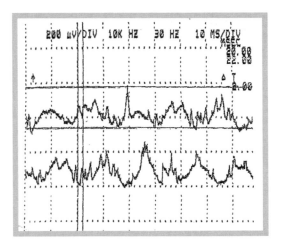

Figure 22

Severe cases require endotracheal intubation and mechanically assisted ventilation, as well as a parenteral hyperalimentation for up to several weeks. In the absence of cerebral hypoxemia, recovery is usually complete.

Acute epiglottitis

Fulminant infection of the epiglottis and arytenoid folds were previously caused almost exclusively by *Haemophilus influenzae* type b (Hib). The clinical course is frequently complicated by abrupt airway obstruction requiring immediate tracheostomy or endotracheal intubation for survival. Hypoxic brain damage or death will occur in a significant number of patients if infection is not recognized.

An autopsy specimen, taken from a boy who died when hospitalization, intravenous antibiotics and observation were the standard of care, had an edematous and infected epiglottis and arytenoid folds. In anticipation of such a complication, 'prophylactic' tracheostomy was proposed in the early 1970s.

Figure 23 shows an erythematous, edematous epiglottis in a child with epiglottitis who required tracheostomy for abrupt airway obstruction. By the mid-1970s, prophylactic endotracheal intubation to secure the

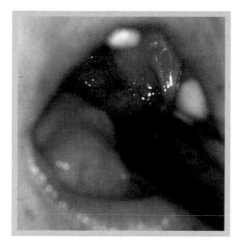

Figure 23

airway had become the standard of care for patients with acute Hib epiglottitis.

This disease has now virtually disappeared with the use of Hib protein-conjugate vaccines, introduced in the late 1980s.

Bacterial meningitis

The clinical presentation of bacterial meningitis may only include fever, irritability or other findings indicating toxicity. The most suggestive physical feature is nuchal rigidity or a positive Brudzinski sign, elicited by rapid flexing of the neck with the child supine, hips and knees extended. With inflammation of the meninges, the patient will involuntarily flex the thigh and knees (Figure 24).

A less sensitive physical finding is the Kernig sign, which is positive when extension of the flexed knee elicits increased pain and crying. The infant in Figure 24 also has preseptal cellulitis, which is highly suggestive of *Haemophilus influenzae* as the etiology. In almost all cases of preseptal or orbital cellulitis associated with meningitis, meningeal signs are present during the initial presentation. On rare occasions, however, they may not be apparent until 24 h after beginning treatment.

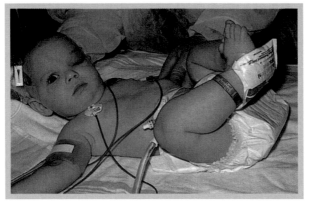

Figure 24

A Gram stain of CSF should always be performed for early identification of etiology, as this may influence the selection of initial antimicrobial therapy and decisions for adding dexamethasome during early treatment. The most common pathogens in infants and children are *Streptococcus pneumoniae* and *Neisseria meningitidis*. Group B streptococci remain the most common cause of meningitis in neonates, followed by *Escherichia coli* and *Listeria monocytogenes*. In fatal cases, gross purulence of the brain is seen at postmortem examination.

Recurrent bacterial meningitis

Recurrent episodes of meningitis necessitate a careful search for cranial and mid-line defects as predisposing factors. Plain radiography and tomography may detect only large defects, and dye or radioisotope tracer studies using nasal packs only occasionally detect CSF leaks. Cranial CT using coronal thin-section views of the anterior cranial fossa (Figure 25) allows detailed examination of the most likely region to have an anatomical defect.

Coronal CT of the anterior cranial fossa indicates an osseous defect in the cribriform plate. Figure 26 is a CT of the anterior cranial fossa showing a unilateral defect in the cribriform plate with soft tissue protrusion into the ethmoid area.

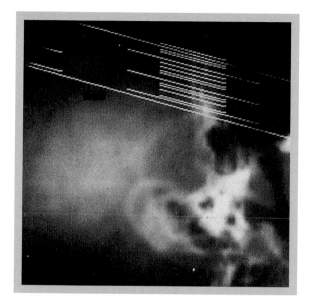

Figure 25

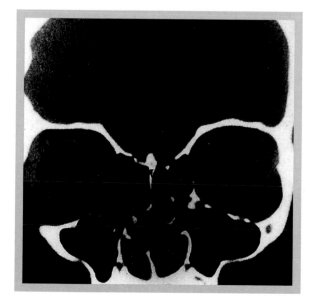

Figure 26

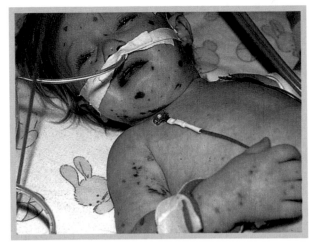

Figure 27

Meningococcemia

Neisseria meningitidis causes illness in humans with a variety of clinical presentations, ranging from benign upper respiratory infection to acute endotoxemia. Vasculitis and chronic disease are also described. The common signs and symptoms of acute and chronic meningococcemia may initially be subtle, but fever accompanied by an ecchymotic, petechial or purpuric rash (Figure 27) should always suggest this diagnosis.

Ecchymoses or purpura are defined as non-blanching skin lesions generally measuring 2–10 mm. The rash may be more petechial (lesions 1–2 mm), particularly with chronic disease. Lesions measuring > 10 mm are associated with a poor prognosis. Disseminated intravascular coagulation and large vessel thrombosis may necessitate extensive amputation.

Diagnosis of meningococcemia is made by a characteristic, clinical presentation and is usually confirmed by culture. Care must be taken to differentiate meningococcemia from other febrile illnesses with rashes. These include septicemia due to other bacteria (particularly

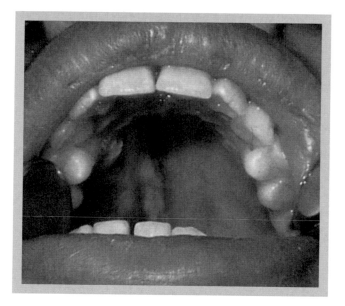

Figure 28

pneumococcus and staphylococcus), endocarditis, Rocky Mountain spotted fever and enteroviral infections.

Treatment of meningococcemia includes antibiotics and intensive supportive care when shock is present. In addition, prophylactic treatment of family members and other close contacts of the index case is indicated, using rifampin, ciprofloxacin or, for pregnant women, ceftriaxone.

Mucormycosis

Acute rhinocerebral mucormycosis is diagnosed most frequently in patients with insulin-dependent diabetes or immunodeficiency and has a high mortality. Illness begins with pain, swelling and tenderness at the site of primary infection. Necrotic lesions appear in the nasal cavity or palate (Figure 28). Hemorrhage into these lesions results in a characteristic black discoloration (not seen in this patient).

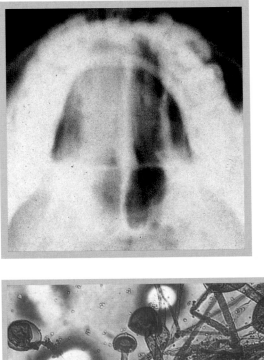

Figure 29

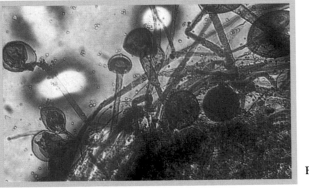

Figure 30

Infection may rapidly destroy bone in the sinuses (Figure 29) and extend into the central nervous system. Thrombosis of the cavernous sinus or internal carotid artery may occur.

Diagnosis is made by tissue biopsy showing non-septate, irregularly branching hyphal forms of *Rhizopus oryzae* (Figure 30), *R. rhizopodoformis* or other members of the order Mucorales.

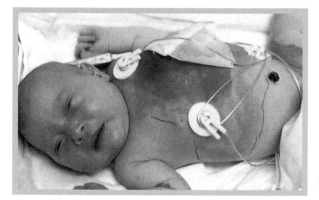

Figure 31

Necrotizing fasciitis

Classification of necrotizing soft tissue infections is based on the anatomical structures involved, the pathogens recovered and the clinical presentation. Bacteriologically, there are two distinct types of necrotizing fasciitis: type I is polymicrobial and involves synergistic interactions among bacteria to produce an aggressive destructive infection; type II is caused by group A beta-hemolytic streptococci alone or in combination with *S. aureus*.

In neonates, *E. coli* is a common single pathogen, as in the infant in Figure 31, whose skin discoloration progressed in just over 5 h from an area measuring 2 x 1 cm to involve the entire chest and abdomen. Treatment is radical surgical debridement of all devitalized tissues (Figure 32) and appropriate antibiotics.

Purpura fulminans

Disseminated intravascular coagulation (DIC) may produce thrombocytopenic purpura with hemorrhagic infection and necrosis of the skin. This often-fatal process is seen most frequently in children and is precipitated by severe infection caused by streptococci, meningococci, varicella-zoster, measles or rickettsiae. In addition, protein C and protein S deficiencies can cause similar disease in neonates.

49

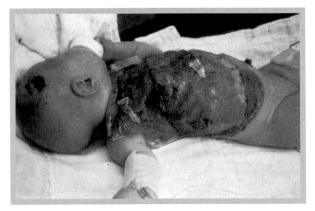

Figure 32

The primary pathology is a consumptive coagulopathy of plasma coagulation factors (fibrinogen factors II, V and VIII) with associated thrombocytopenia, hypofibrinogenemia and hypoprothrombinemia. Even with early treatment of the infection and correction of clotting factor deficiencies, the mortality rate is 20%.

A girl with hemorrhagic chickenpox developed purpura fulminans associated with group A beta-hemolytic streptococcal bacteremia. Her leukocyte count was 50 000/mm³ with a hemoglobin of 6 g/dl. Platelet count was also 50 000/mm³. Recovery was complete following penicillin therapy.

The child in Figure 33 developed DIC with extensive purpura on the 3rd day of sepsis and meningitis caused by *N. meningitidis*. Recovery after penicillin therapy was complete without sequelae.

Staphylococcal toxic shock syndrome (Staph-TSS)

Epidemic staphylococcal toxic shock syndrome occurred in the USA in association with the introduction and use of hyperabsorbable and occlusive vaginal tampons in the late 1980s. These products were withdrawn from the market and the incidence of menstruation-associated disease decreased dramatically. However, sporadic cases of menstrual- and non-menstrual-associated staphylococcal toxic shock syndrome continue to be reported.

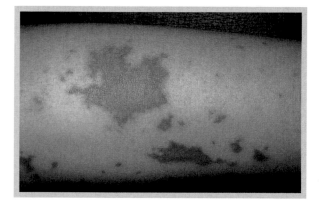

Figure 33

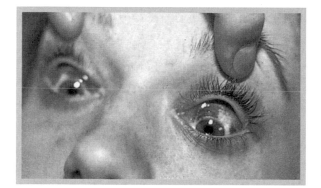

Figure 34

The site of infection is usually superficial. There is a characteristic prodrome of high fever, headache, sore throat, abdominal pain and severe vomiting with watery diarrhea. This is followed by increasing toxicity and, after 24–48 h, by marked non-suppurative conjunctival injection, often with hemorrhage (Figure 34), with hyperemia of the oral mucosa and hypertrophy of the papilla of the tongue (Figure 35) similar to that seen in scarlet fever and Kawasaki syndrome. This is soon followed by a sunburn-like erythematous macular rash, which usually starts on the trunk and becomes generalized.

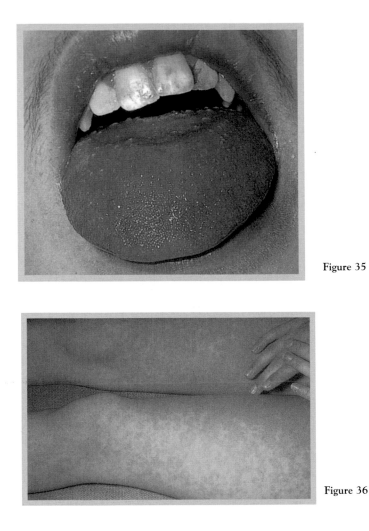

Figure 35

Figure 36

Figure 36 shows erythroderma and delayed capillary filling. Petechiae occur especially around the wrists and ankles, and shiny edema of the hands and feet (Figure 37) may be seen. Postural hypotension ensues, associated with confusion and lethargy, and followed by shock, multiple organ failure and death in 5–10% of patients if early

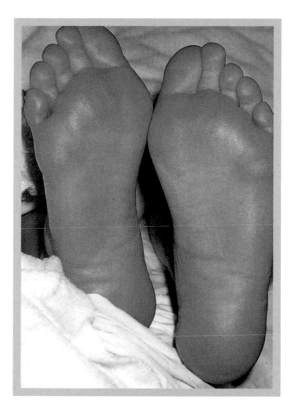

Figure 37

treatment is not provided. Erythroderma fades after 2–4 days, and full-thickness desquamation of the hands (Figure 38) and feet occurs after 1–2 weeks.

Streptococcal toxic shock syndrome (Strep-TSS)

This is caused by toxin-producing strains of invasive group A β-hemolytic streptococci (GABHS). The disease is characterized by a vague prodrome of increasing deep painful swelling and tenderness of an extremity over 2–3 days following injury to the area. Abrupt onset of fever, rigors, toxicity and shock may occur with rapid development of multi-organ failure. Mortality varies from 30 to 50%, primarily due to delay in diagnosis and treatment.

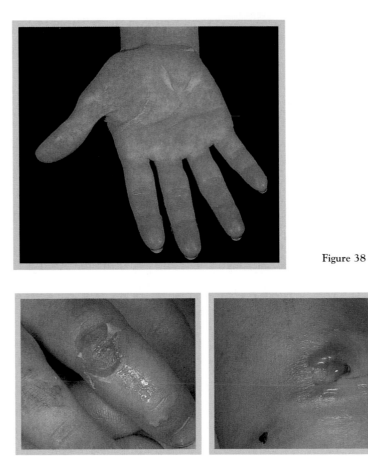

Figure 38

Figure 39   Figure 40

The girl shown in Figure 39 (courtesy of Dr M.E. Weisse) had an abscess on her finger. Four days later (3 days prior to hospitalization), she fell and hurt her right shoulder, producing pain and swelling which persisted for 2 days. Several hours prior to hospital admission, she developed a vesiculobullous lesion in the right antecubital area (Figure 40), high fever, rigors, toxicity, lethargy, shock and cardio-

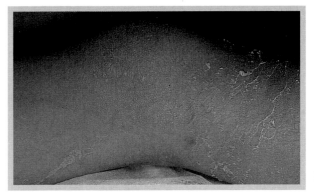

Figure 41

pulmonary arrest. The child was treated with antibiotics, fluid resuscitation, intubation and assisted ventilation. A generalized erythematous rash developed over 24 h and subsided over the next 2–3 days, followed by desquamation 7–10 days later (Figure 41). GABHS was cultured from the blood obtained on admission.

A boy with fever of up to 40.5°C, lasting 12 h, showed a normal initial examination, complete blood count (CBC), urinalysis and chest radiograph. The patient became pallid, then ashen, followed by cardiopulmonary arrest while being sponged with water to reduce the fever. Intubation, ventilation, fluid resuscitation, ionotropic therapy and parenteral antibiotics were provided, but the child remained anuric with poor cardiac output. Left lower lobe pneumonia with effusion developed over several hours and a Gram stain of the pleural fluid showed Gram-positive cocci in chains. GABHS grew on culture. The child developed multiple organ failure including shock-lung, and died 18 h after hospital admission (30 h after onset of illness).

Maculopapular exanthematous diseases

Drug eruptions

Antibiotics, analgesics, anticonvulsants, and various food substitutes and flavorings are often implicated as causing allergic skin rashes in children. Fixed drug eruptions characteristically recur in the same site and are discrete oval or round infiltrative lesions, varying from 0.5 to several centimeters in size. Purpura with vesicles and/or bullae may be seen. Pruritus is minimal or absent. Lesions persist for 1–3 weeks with spontaneous resolution after removal of the offending agent.

The fixed drug eruption in a child shown in Figure 42 was due to clindamycin and/or ampicillin, which had been taken on several occasions. A similar rash had been observed 1 year previously.

Phenytoin is associated with a particularly high incidence of drug eruptions. The child in Figure 43 presented with a pruritic maculopapular scarlatiniform generalized eruption of 11 days' duration. Persistent fever, sore throat, generalized lymphadenopathy and aphthous mouth ulcers were found. CBC showed leukocytosis with 43% atypical lymphocytes.

Enteroviral infections

Enteroviruses, a subgroup of picornaviruses, are a common cause of exanthems in children. These viruses (poliovirus, coxsackievirus, echovirus and reovirus) spread by contact from person to person, and initiate infection in the oropharynx before attacking the gastro-intestinal tract. The rash is usually generalized, non-pruritic and maculopapular, but may be vesicular, scarlatiniform, zosteriform,

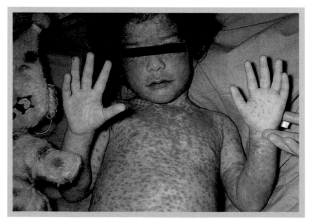

Figure 42

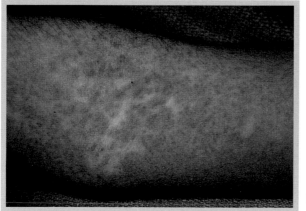

Figure 43

urticarial, petechial or purpuric. The majority of these eruptions persist for 2–8 days.

A typical example of the pruritic maculopapular eruption is shown in Figure 44 in a child who had no other symptoms. No medications had been taken. Examination was normal except for the generalized rash that was also on the palms and soles. The rash cleared spontaneously in 8 days.

The enanthem in Figure 45, characterized by aphthous ulcers on the soft palate (herpangina), in a teenager with a generalized maculopapular rash, fever, sore throat and tender anterior cervical lymph nodes is most compatible with coxsackie A virus infection.

Epstein–Barr virus

The infectious mononucleosis syndrome characterized by fever, sore throat, fatigue, malaise and generalized lymphadenopathy is associated with Epstein–Barr virus (EBV), although adenovirus, CMV, *Toxoplasma gondii*, viral hepatitis, HIV and drug hypersensitivity may occasionally produce a similar illness.

A previously healthy child developed fever, a generalized papular rash, sore throat, dysphagia, arthralgia and abdominal pain.

57

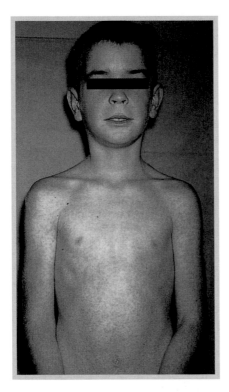

Figure 44

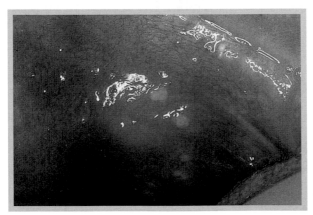

Figure 45

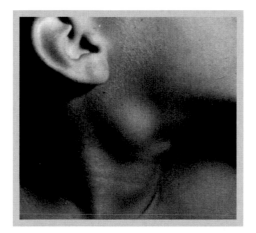

Figure 46

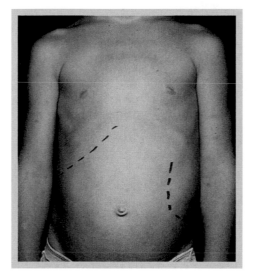

Figure 47

Lymphadenopathy (Figure 46), hepatosplenomegaly (Figure 47) and exudative tonsillitis were noted. CBC showed 34 000 leukocytes/mm³ with 37% atypical lymphocytes and abundant cytoplasm (Downey cells; Figure 48). A monospot test was positive and a four-fold rise in

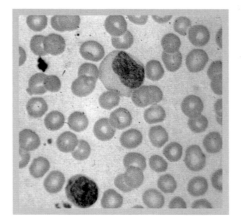

Figure 48

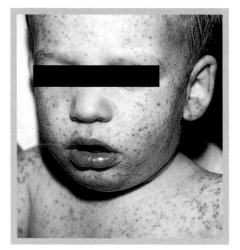

Figure 49

EBV-specific serology confirmed the diagnosis. Spontaneous recovery occurred within 3 weeks.

In a younger patient, amoxicillin for 3 days was ineffective and, in fact, accentuated the rash into a widespread pustular dermatitis (Figure 49). Note the eyelid edema and petechiae on the ear lobes, both of which are characteristic of infectious mononucleosis.

EBV infection may also cause a spectrum of oncological processes, such as Burkitt's lymphoma, nasopharyngeal carcinoma, Hodgkin's disease and lymphoproliferative disorders, especially in patients with immunodeficient states and/or AIDS.

Erythema infectiosum

Parvovirus B19 infection in children usually presents as a mild exanthematous illness, termed erythema infectiosum (also called fifth disease). It begins with a distinctive 'slapped cheek' red rash lasting 1–3 days, followed by a generalized maculopapular exanthem of 7–10 days' duration. The rash may increase in intensity, producing a lace-like appearance, during periods of increased physical activity, exposure to sunlight or high environmental temperatures. Fever occurs in 15–30% of patients during the first 2 days of illness, and arthralgia is common in adult women.

Parvovirus B19 infection may also produce a mild respiratory illness, arthritis in adults, chronic anemia in immunodeficient patients, an aplastic crisis in patients with chronic hemolytic anemias, and severe anemia with hydrops fetalis in the fetus of an infected pregnant woman.

The child in Figure 50 presented with a fever and non-pruritic rash for 2 days. The cheeks were intensely red and a diffuse maculopapular rash persisted for 10 days. During the next 3–4 weeks, a transient lace-like rash (Figure 51) was noted for several hours during increased physical activity.

Erythema multiforme minor

Erythema multiforme (EM) is a distinct hypersensitivity syndrome of unknown pathogenesis, characterized by unique skin and mucous membrane lesions. Infectious agents are the most common precipitating etiologies. EM can be differentiated from urticaria by the primary skin lesions. In EM, all lesions appear within 72 h and remain in a fixed location for at least 7 days. Papules, usually totaling over 100, evolve into target lesions with central vesicles, bullae or crusts. Itching or burning of individual lesions occurs, but is rarely severe.

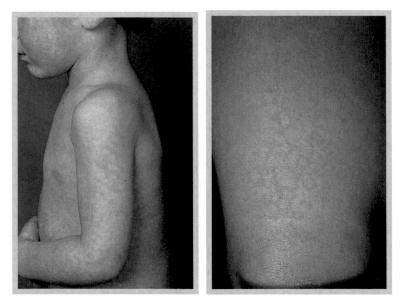

Figure 50   **Figure 51**

EM due to coxsackie A virus was diagnosed in a teenager with a 6-day history of a generalized pruritic erythematous rash, and tender mouth and hands. Tetracycline had been taken for 4 days and 'allergy pills' for 2 days. Examination was normal except for multiple fixed iris and circular macules, with central target red–purple lesions particularly concentrated on the extremities. Vesicopustules were seen in the mouth and on the fingers (Figure 52), ankles and feet. Spontaneous resolution occurred within 2 weeks.

Kawasaki disease

Because there is no definitive laboratory test to identify Kawasaki disease, diagnosis depends on the presence of fever lasting longer than 5 days plus four of the five following clinical features (Figure 53):

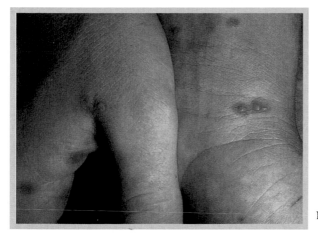

Figure 52

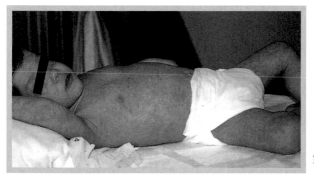

Figure 53

(1)   Bulbar conjunctivitis;

(2)   An enanthem of erythematous mouth and pharynx, strawberry tongue and red cracked lips;

(3)   A generalized erythematous rash;

(4)   Extremity changes, such as swelling or erythema;

(5)   Adenopathy, with one cervical node > 1.5 cm in diameter.

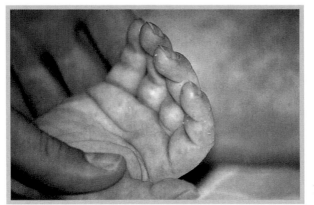

Figure 54

Other features include sterile pyuria, arthritis, arthralgia, carditis and gallbladder hydrops. Following the acute phase, desquamation of the fingertips (Figure 54) or hands and feet is characteristic. Coronary aneurysms represent the most serious consequence of this disease (Figure 55) as death may result from occlusion subsequent to thrombus formation or progressive artery stenosis. High-dose intravenous immunoglobulin, in conjunction with aspirin, decreases the incidence of coronary artery disease.

Measles

Rubeola or measles begins with a prodrome of increasing fever, clear rhinorrhea, photophobia and cough of 2–5 days' duration. A rash then develops on the face along the forehead and in front of the ears, and soon involves the whole of the face, with conjunctival injection. Rhinorrhea and cough worsen and there may be epiphora.

Koplik spots appear on the buccal mucosa opposite the upper and lower premolar teeth (Figure 56) 24–48 h before onset of the rash, and may persist for 48–72 h after onset of the rash. If the spots are not present 24 h before and after onset of the rash, then diagnosis of measles is unlikely.

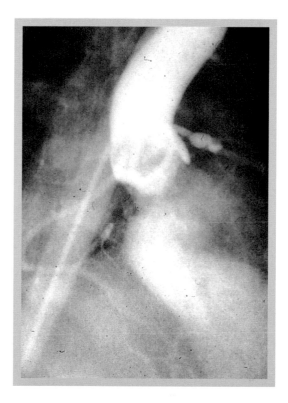

Figure 55

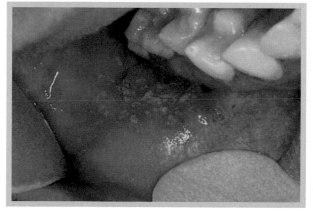

Figure 56

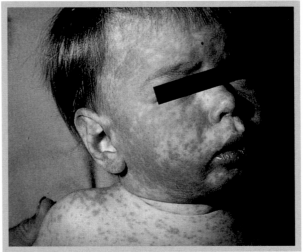

Figure 57

On the first day of the rash, reddish-purple macules 3–7 mm in diameter coalesce on the face and shoulders to become confluent (Figure 57). On the second day, the rash appears on the shoulders and trunk and, by the third day, spreads to the thighs. At this time, the rash on the face fades, leaving a fine white powdery desquamation. Fever and rhinorrhea subside, but the cough persists for 1–2 weeks.

Patients who received killed measles virus vaccine when it was available during 1963–1968 are only partially protected. Once exposed to the natural virus, the disease assumes an atypical presentation (atypical measles), with a centrifugal maculopapular to petechial rash (Figures 58 and 59) following a prodrome of high fever, headache, abdominal pain and myalgia. A non-productive cough associated with pleuritic chest pain is commonly seen as a consequence of pneumonia and often with a pleural effusion. Evolution of the rash is variable. Only the distal extremities are involved in some patients whereas, in others, the trunk as well as the entire extremities are affected. Patients with atypical measles are not considered contagious.

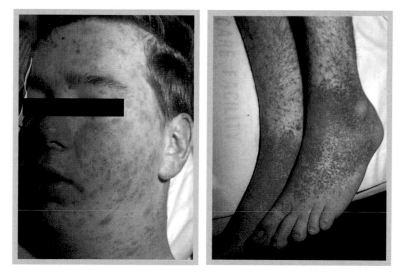

Figure 58   **Figure 59**

Roseola infantum

Human herpesvirus 6 (HHV-6) was first isolated in 1986 from cultures of patients with lymphoreticular disease. This herpesvirus group is ubiquitous. By 3 years of age, most children have been infected. HHV-6 has two subgroups: A and B. No disease is presently associated with group A whereas group B appears to be the major etiological agent of roseola, also called sixth disease or exanthem subitum.

Infection is characterized by 3–5 days of high fever with a paucity of physical findings. The temperature rapidly returns to normal, at which time a morbilliform rash appears. Figure 60 demonstrates roseola, where rash was preceded by 3 days of temperatures up to 104°F and irritability, but otherwise normal findings on physical examination. On the fourth day, the patient was afebrile with an extensive generalized maculopapular rash and bilateral 10 -mm suboccipital nodes. The rash faded within 48 h.

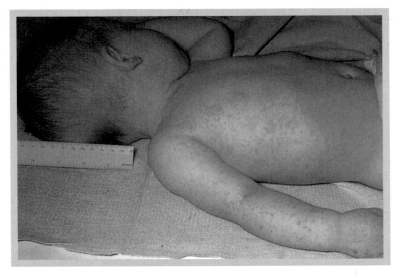

Figure 60

Rubella

Rubella, a togavirus, usually causes a mild 3-day illness. Clinical features are minimal with low-grade fever, a fine discrete maculopapular rash and generalized lymphadenopathy, particularly postauricular, suboccipital cervical and/or suboccipital. Transient polyarthralgia and polyarthritis occasionally occur in children, but are common in female adolescents and adults. Encephalitis and thrombocytopenia are rare complications.

The child in Figure 61 developed low-grade fever and non-pruritic generalized, discrete, maculopapular eruption, which resolved spontaneously within 72 h. Another child of the same age also had postauricular adenopathy (Figure 62).

Scarlet fever

Scarlet fever occurs with pharyngitis or wound infections due to erythrogenic toxins produced by GABHS. The rash starts on the

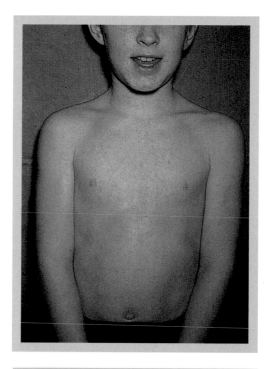

Figure 61

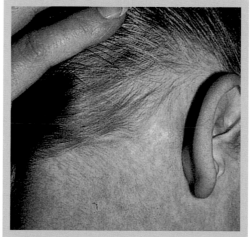

Figure 62

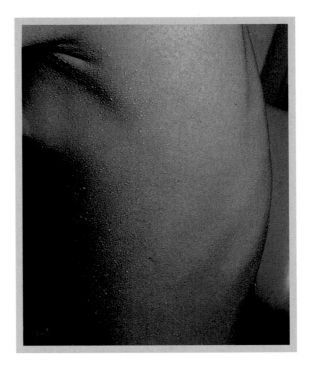

Figure 63

neck, axillae and shoulders, and is usually faint on the face, where a malar flush with circumoral pallor may be more evident.

The rash is most pronounced on the trunk, appearing as a generalized sunburn-like erythroderma (Figure 63). There is a palpable sandpaper-like texture to the skin in involved areas due to hypertrophy of the openings of the sweat and sebaceous glands.

The hallmark of the rash of scarlet fever is the marked intensity of the rash in the flexural creases; this is most apparent in the axillae and groin (Figure 64), but is also seen in the antecubital areas where the darkened creases are called Pastia lines (Figure 65). The erythroderma begins to fade after 2–3 days and a generalized desquamation, starting

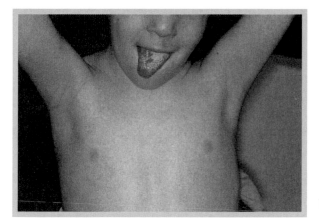

Figure 64

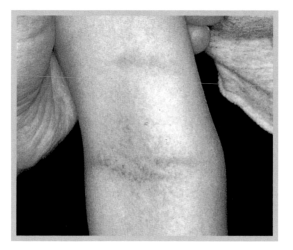

Figure 65

with the hands (Figure 66) and feet, occurs after 7–10 days. (Figures 63–66 are courtesy of Dr M.E. Weisse.)

Staphylococcal scalded skin syndrome (SSSS)

This term refers to a spectrum of dermatological disorders caused by a soluble exotoxin produced by certain strains of *Staphylococcus aureus*.

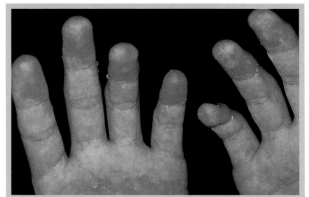

Figure 66

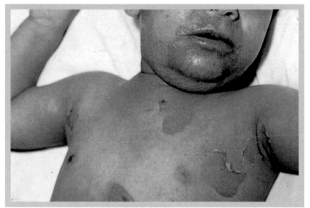

Figure 67

Disease is most severe in neonates, termed Ritter's disease, in which there is a bullous desquamation of large areas of skin. More common is a diffuse scarlatiniform erythroderma, which progresses to desquamation of involved areas and a positive Nikolsky sign (Figure 67).

In the USA, most of the exotoxin-producing staphylococci belong to phage group II. The characteristic histopathological feature is a cleavage plane high in the epidermis with no inflammatory reaction.

Papulovesicular exanthematous diseases

Coxsackievirus infections

Human enteroviruses include 23 which are classified as coxsackie A viruses and six which are coxsackie B. In infants and young children, these viruses usually produce illnesses which are non-specific and febrile. Other less common, but more serious, diseases are seen in the summer and fall, and involve one of the following organ systems:

(1) Upper and lower respiratory tract: common cold, pharyngitis, herpangina, stomatitis, pneumonia and pleurodynia;

(2) Gastrointestinal: vomiting, diarrhea, abdominal pain and hepatitis;

(3) Eye: acute hemorrhagic conjunctivitis;

(4) Heart: myopericarditis;

(5) Skin: exanthems;

(6) Neurological: aseptic meningitis, encephalitis and paralysis.

Figure 68 shows coxsackievirus A9 infection, with fever, severe sore throat, multiple oropharyngeal vesicopustular lesions, and a

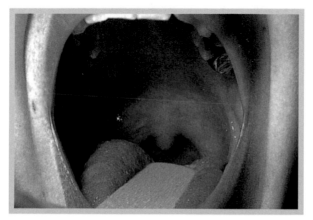

Figure 68

73

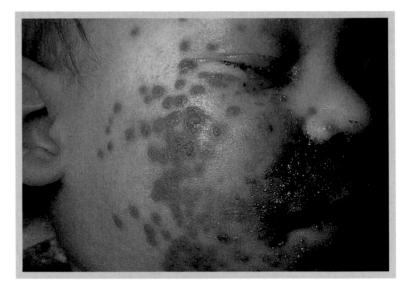

Figure 69

maculopapular rash of the head, neck and trunk. Spontaneous recovery occurred within 6 days.

Coxsackievirus A5 causes illness with malaise, headache, coryza, fever, generalized adenopathy, hepatosplenomegaly and a maculopapular rash. The rash becomes papulovesicular on day 5, but resolves spontaneously with fine desquamation and complete recovery by day 7.

Eczema herpeticum

Cutaneous dissemination of HSV type 1 and 2 in patients with atopic eczema or chronic dermatitis is termed eczema herpeticum or Kaposi varicelliform eruption. Figure 69 shows an example of extensive HSV infection on the face with atopic dermatitis. The HSV dermatitis cleared spontaneously within 14 days without treatment.

The disease is variable, ranging from mild self-limiting lesions to rapidly fatal infection. Extensive vesicular and crusting eruptions may

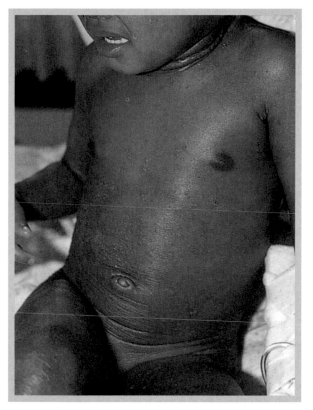

Figure 70

result in painful weeping, with excessive fluid loss and bacterial superinfection (Figure 70). Patients usually have high fever and are irritable.

Severe manifestations are associated with deficient cell-mediated immunity, such as in the Wiskott–Aldrich syndrome. In limited trials, both intravenous and oral acyclovir has been shown to control progression of the disease. The differential diagnosis includes eczema with secondary bacterial infection and varicella.

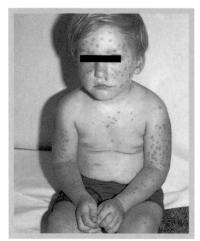

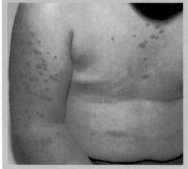

Figure 72

Figure 71

Gianotti–Crosti syndrome

Also known as papular acrodermatitis of childhood, this disease is characterized by the rapid development of symmetrical flat-topped (lichenoid) skin-colored or erythematous papules in a centrifugal distribution (Figures 71 and 72). It is self-limiting, but lasts for 3–6 weeks.

One-quarter of these cases are associated with hepatitis B, as in the child in Figure 71 who had hepatomegaly, elevation of liver enzymes and positive serology for hepatitis B surface antigen. Most cases in children are anicteric. Outbreaks have been reported with EBV infection and case reports suggest that this rash is also a manifestation of AIDS.

Other viral agents that produce this rash include parainfluenza and coxsackie A16 viruses. The peak age of incidence is 1–6 years with a 2 : 1 male to female predominance. These cutaneous changes are presumed to be a reaction to either viral or immune complex deposition.

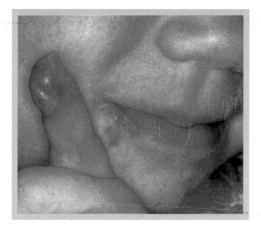

Figure 73

Herpetic whitlow

Primary cutaneous herpes may be found anywhere, but is particularly common in children who suck their thumbs or fingers, with inoculation and as a secondary infection of the digits. The lesion is a painful vesicular eruption. Where the diagnosis is not clinically apparent, Tzanck test preparations, fluorescent staining for herpes or viral cultures may be performed on scrapings of the lesions. Figure 73 shows herpetic whitlow in a child with recurrent herpes simplex labialis.

Impetigo

This term refers to superficial infection of the skin that may be primary or secondary to abrasions and insect bites. Impetigo lesions are classified as pustular, honey-crusted (Figure 74) or bullous (Figure 75). The latter is due almost exclusively to *Staphylococcus aureus*. Prior to 1980, impetigo was caused primarily by GABHS and, although *S. aureus* was also frequently implicated, treatment with penicillin alone was sufficient. Subsequently, however, penicillin-resistant *S. aureus* has evolved as the major cause of impetigo. An oral macrolide, a penicillinase-resistant penicillin, a cephalosporin or a topical antibiotic provide optimal treatment.

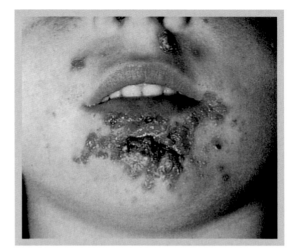

Figure 74

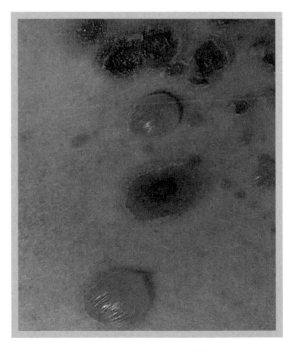

Figure 75

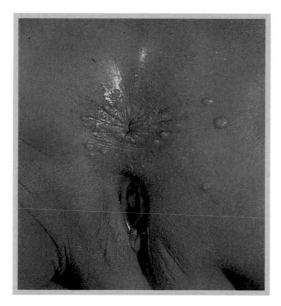

Figure 76

Molluscum contagiosum

Poxvirus infection of the skin is manifested by single or multiple raised, firm, smooth, waxy, skin-colored, flat or umbilicated tumors, which vary in size from one to several millimeters in diameter. These lesions occur primarily in children and tend to resolve spontaneously over several months. Numerous molluscum lesions in the anogenital area (Figure 76) may be the result of child abuse.

Papular urticaria

This common childhood eruption is a sensitivity reaction to insects such as fleas, mosquitoes and chiggers. Children usually present in the spring or summer with multiple bites and/or papules and wheals on all extremities and, to a lesser extent, on the face, trunk and buttocks.

The rash comprises numerous urticated papules 3–10 mm in diameter with occasional wheals, some with a central hemorrhagic punctum. Because pruritus is usually present, scratching produces secondary

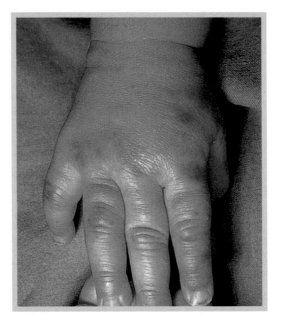

Figure 77

excoriation, inflammatory ulcerations and impetiginized crusts. If insect bites are subsequently avoided, most lesions resolve within 10–21 days, but may persist for months or even years if the child is re-exposed to insect bites.

The child shown in Figure 77 presented with pruritic papules and wheals on all extremities for several days. The mother noted a daily variation in the intensity of the rash from one extremity to another. Examination revealed multiple purpuric and inflamed papules and wheals on all extremities, and similar lesions on the face. The family dog was treated for fleas and the infant treated with diphenhydramine. The rash resolved within 17 days.

Another child presented with a similar history of multiple inflamed papules and wheals on all extremities. Pruritus was moderate. All lesions resolved within 2 weeks with diphenhydramine therapy and elimination of cat fleas.

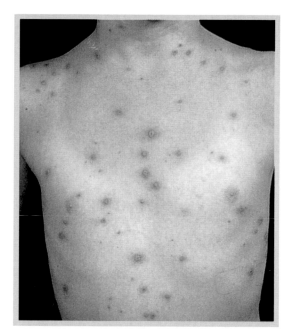

Figure 78

Varicella-zoster

Primary varicella is referred to as chickenpox, whereas exacerbation of latent infection is termed herpes zoster or shingles. Varicella lesions first appear on the face and along the hairline, then spread to the trunk within 1–2 days (Figure 78).

Although varicella skin lesions vary in form from erythematous macules to papules, vesicles and pustules, the classic diagnostic lesion is the uniloculated vesicle on an erythematous base, also described as a 'dew-drop on a rose petal'. Crops of macules, papules and pustules are all frequently seen in the same area at the same time, and continue to evolve and resolve over several days into desquamating scales and scabs.

Fever and systemic symptoms vary with the severity of the rash, but most patients have only a few skin lesions, and are afebrile and

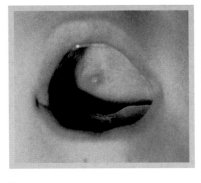

Figure 79

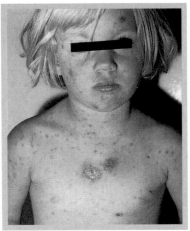

Figure 80

asymptomatic. Approximately one-quarter have an enanthem which is manifested as ulcerative lesions on the oral mucosa (Figure 79).

The most common complication of varicella is secondary infection of the lesions, most often due to GABHS (Figure 80). Although apparently trivial, these infections may progress to severe invasive disease (see streptococcal toxic shock syndrome).

Herpes zoster usually occurs in subjects with a history of mild varicella at a young age or where previous infection was subclinical. It begins with hyperesthesia or pain along a neurocutaneous pathway on the trunk (Figure 81) or on a branch of the trigeminal nerve. The lesions typically appear in clusters of vesicles on an erythematous base, arranged in a linear dermatone distribution.

Enanthems

Candidiasis

Thrush is the common term used to describe oral candidiasis, manifested by the presence of irregular white plaques on the tongue,

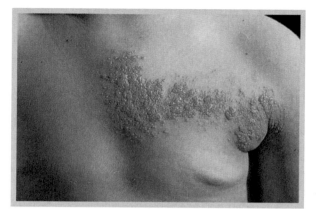

Figure 81

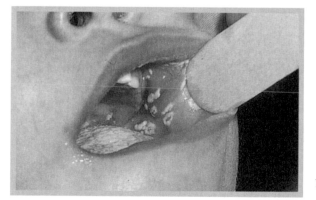

Figure 82

buccal mucosa, lips and palate (Figure 82). Gram staining shows large Gram-positive budding yeast with pseudohyphae.

The peak incidence of thrush occurs in infants during the first 2–3 months of life but may be seen in otherwise healthy children up to 1 year of age. Candidiasis may also be seen in older children who have been treated with broad-spectrum antibiotics. Severe and persistent oral candidiasis suggests an underlying immunodeficiency.

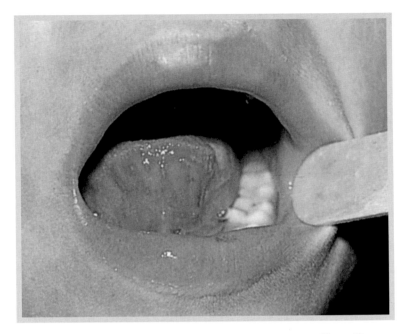

Figure 83

Cyclic neutropenia

Defective maturation of uncommitted stem white blood cells results in an absolute neutropenia that may be cyclical. Clinically, this is manifested as episodic fever, aphthous stomatitis (Figure 83), cervical lymphadenitis and gastroenteritis occurring at relatively regular intervals, every 3–6 weeks.

Signs and symptoms are usually not evident until the neutrophil count has already begun to rise. Diagnosis therefore requires quantitation of white blood cell concentrations in blood during the period immediately preceding the anticipated clinical events. Some patients may also have similar cyclical fluctuations in erythrocytes and platelets.

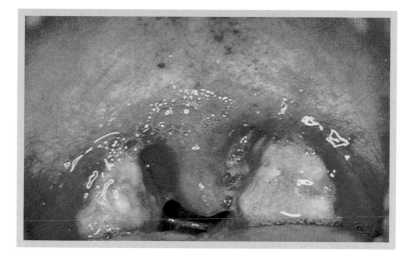

Figure 84

Treatment includes aggressive oral hygiene, antibiotics during febrile or symptomatic episodes and granulocyte colony-stimulating factor (G-CSF) for more severe infectious complications.

Exudative tonsillopharyngitis

Most upper respiratory tract infections are caused by viral agents and require only symptomatic therapy, as in the teenager in Figure 84 whose pharyngitis was caused by EBV. Note the petechiae on the soft palate. As pharyngitis or tonsillitis without nasal involvement is more commonly associated with group A streptococci, a throat culture test for streptococcal antigen is essential for determining bacterial etiology. Often, documentation of an outbreak of oropharyngeal infection caused by a particular viral pathogen will provide guidance to the management of subsequent cases.

Rare, but important, bacterial pathogens that cause pharyngitis are *Arcanobacterium hemolyticum*, *N. gonorrhoeae*, *Corynebacterium*

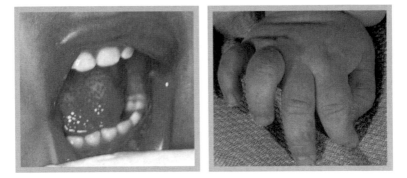

Figure 85   Figure 86

diphtheriae and *Francisella tularensis*, with other groups of streptococci, particularly C and G, accounting for isolated outbreaks of disease.

Hand–foot–mouth disease

Coxsackieviruses A16, A5, A9, A10, B1 and B3 may produce a low-grade fever, headache and vesicular lesions in the mouth, hands and feet which last for 3–10 days, occasionally with associated aseptic meningitis. The mouth lesions are yellowish ulcers with erythematous borders on the tongue, lips, gums, buccal mucosa and palate (Figure 85). Skin lesions comprise erythematous macules, papules and vesicles on the hands (Figure 86) and feet (Figure 87) and, less commonly, on the buttocks. Lesions on the hands and feet are oval, with the long axis lying parallel to the dermal ridges. Some lesions may appear pustular.

Hand–foot–mouth disease should be differentiated from primary herpetic gingivostomatitis in which gingivitis, fever and cervical lymphadenopathy are prominent.

Herpangina

One or more oral yellowish ulcers several millimeters in diameter, with surrounding erythematous rings measuring an additional 4–6 mm in diameter, are characteristic of herpangina. Lesions are most often seen

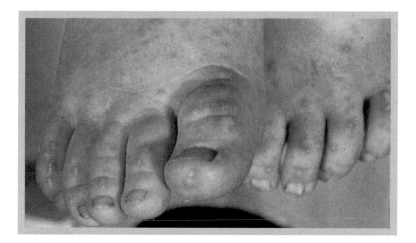

Figure 87

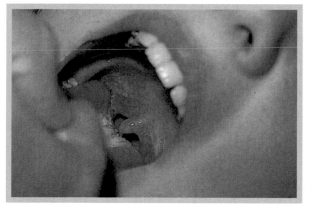

Figure 88

on the anterior tonsillar pillar (Figure 88), less often on the uvula and soft palate, and rarely on the posterior pharyngeal wall. Lesions are not seen anterior to these areas. There may be mild-to-moderate fever, sore throat, irritability and feeding difficulty in young infants, and headache and malaise in older children.

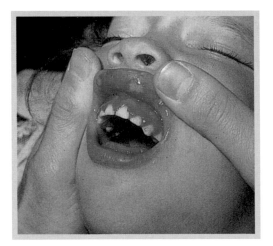

Figure 89

Herpangina is caused by infection by a number of coxsackieviruses (both A and B) and by echoviruses. The disease usually lasts only 3–6 days. Some cases may have associated aseptic meningitis.

Herpes gingivostomatitis

Primary herpetic gingivostomatitis (PHGS) occurs in children aged between 6 months and 3 years who present with yellowish ulcers that are one to several millimeters in diameter on the gums, gingiva, buccal mucosa, lips, tongue and palate, most with surrounding rings of erythema (Figure 89). The lesions are not seen in the posterior mouth or pharynx, but there may be a preceding exudative tonsillo-pharyngitis without mouth lesions, particularly in older children and adults.

The gingiva are frequently edematous with a purplish erythema, and are tender, painful and friable with a tendency to bleed when touched. In older children who are thumb-suckers, PHGS may be associated with secondary herpetic whitlow (Figure 90).

Most children with PHGS have mild-to-moderate fever and anterior cervical lymphadenopathy. The disease usually lasts only 4–7 days, but

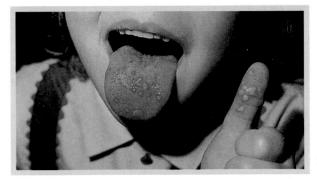

Figure 90

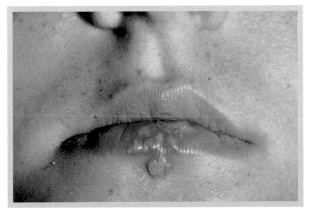

Figure 91

may persist for 1–2 weeks. Some foods and juices may cause pain when taken, but most children are able to take milk and milk products, including ice cream, to maintain adequate hydration and nutrition.

As the primary infection subsides, the virus establishes a latent infection in the trigeminal ganglia for life and may express exacerbation as recurrent herpes labialis infections or 'fever blisters' (Figure 91).

89

Recurrent aphthae

Single or multiple shallow ulcers which periodically develop on the gums, tongue, palate, oropharynx and buccal mucosa opposite the biting surface of the teeth (Figure 92) are variously called recurrent aphthae, aphthous stomatitis, or aphthae. The term aphthous stomatitis has also been used synonymously with herpetic gingivostomatitis.

The cause of aphthae is likely to be minor oral trauma with subsequent bacterial overgrowth, as lesions are more common in children fitted with braces or other orthodontic devices. With chronic trauma, the lesions may form fibrosing mucoceles (Figure 93) adjacent to the ducts of minor salivary glands.

Treatment is rarely necessary except when lesions are extensive or severe. Light cauterization with silver nitrate is advocated by many dermatologists, but aggressive cauterization can result in significant damage to the mucosa (Figure 94).

Stevens–Johnson syndrome

Erythema multiforme major or Stevens–Johnson syndrome is a severe bullous form of erythema that presents with acute onset of high fever and pronounced systematic symptoms. Two or more mucous membranes, usually the mouth and eyes, are initially involved with lesions, followed by the genitalia, perineal and nares.

Stevens–Johnson syndrome lasts 2–6 weeks, depending on the causative agent, which is usually infectious (HSV, EBV, measles virus, Mycoplasma) or drugs (anticonvulsants, sulfonamides, non-steroidal anti-inflammatory drugs). HSV infection accounts for 80% of childhood cases. Ocular changes (keratitis, uveitis, severe conjunctivitis, corneal ulceration, panophthalmitis) may result in partial or complete blindness. Photophobia may be severe and persistent. A mortality of 5% is reported in children, in contrast to 15% in adolescents and adults.

Stevens–Johnson syndrome due to Mycoplasma pneumoniae occurred in the child in Figure 95 who developed cough and coryza for several

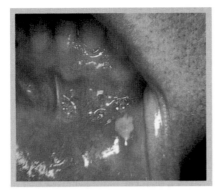

Figure 92

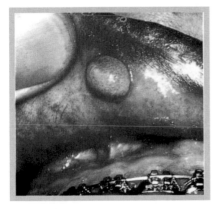

Figure 93

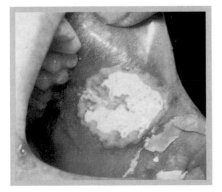

Figure 94

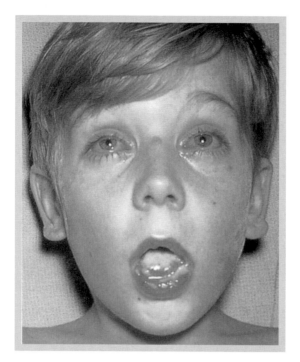

Figure 95

days, followed by acute onset fever, malaise, severe cough and headache. Multiple target lesions appeared rapidly over the trunk and extremities, with severe conjunctivitis and exudative dermatitis of the lips, tongue and, subsequently, the entire oral cavity. Chest X-ray revealed bilateral pneumonitis. Oral erythromycin therapy effected a prompt decrease in fever, cough and malaise, leading to complete recovery after 11 days.

One child developed an extensive generalized erythematous dermatitis with high fever, malaise, anorexia, photophobia, exudative stomatitis and conjunctivitis 10 days after measles was diagnosed. The rash progressed rapidly over 12 h to multiple vesiculobullae, with pruritus and extensive peeling of the skin. In spite of high-dose prednisone therapy (60 mg/day), there was generalized desquamation

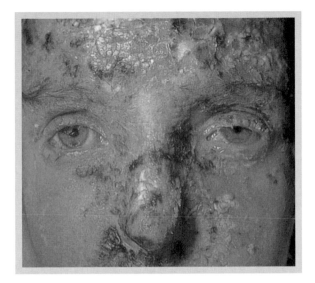

Figure 96

with continuation of fever and malaise. Oral and ocular lesions persisted with severe stomatitis, conjunctivitis and photophobia. By day 18, the skin was healing, but corneal clouding, thinning and corneal ulcerations developed (Figure 96). Over the next 6 weeks, the disease slowly resolved. After 2 months, the skin and oral mucosa were normal. However, the patient had persistent keratitis and photophobia with total blindness due to corneal opacification.

Strawberry tongue

The appearance of strawberry tongue (see Figure 64) is associated with scarlet fever. The tongue and oral mucosa are hyperemic, and there is hypertrophy of the papillae of the tongue. There may be a partial white coat which, after 2–3 days, desquamates to leave a raw uncoated 'raspberry tongue'.

Vincent's gingivostomatitis

Gingival infection with necrosis involving the interdental papillae and gums is referred to as acute necrotizing gingivitis, trench mouth or

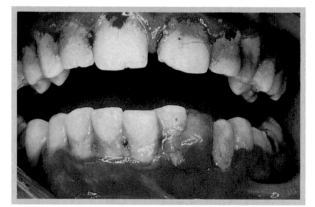

Figure 97

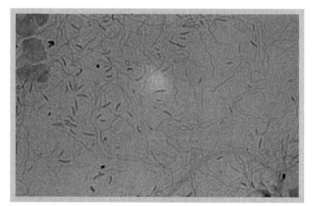

Figure 98

Vincent's gingivostomatitis (Figure 97). When tonsillar tissue is involved, the term 'Vincent's angina' is more appropriate.

The causal organisms are *Borrelia* species (Figure 98) and other penicillin-sensitive fusiform bacilli and spirochetes. In developing countries and historically throughout much of the world, infection was related to malnutrition and poor oral hygiene. Currently, this

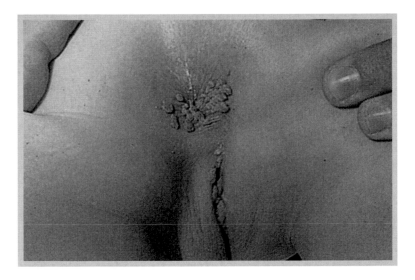

Figure 99

disease is more commonly a consequence of cytolytic chemotherapy in cancer patients, with tissue breakdown in the mouth and secondary overgrowth of colonizing microflora.

Sexually transmitted diseases

Condylomata acuminata

Also known as genital warts, these irregular raised verrucous lesions are often seen on the mucous membranes and mucocutaneous areas of the genitalia and perineal areas (Figure 99), but rarely on the mucous membranes of the mouth. The disease is caused by human papillomaviruses, predominantly types 6 and 11. Incubation may be prolonged so that lesions in infants and children up to 2–3 years of age may have been acquired perinatally. Condylomata acuminata in older children suggests childhood sexual abuse.

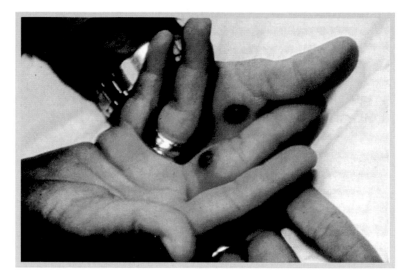

Figure 100

Gonococcal infection

Most uncomplicated gonococcal infections (gonorrhea) produce symptoms of urethritis in adolescent males, whereas disease in females is frequently asymptomatic. Disseminated gonococcal infection following bacteremia often produces petechial or pustular acral skin lesions that begin to appear 3–21 days after exposure, together with asymmetrical arthralgias, tenosynovitis or septic arthritis. This is referred to as the arthritis–dermatitis syndrome (Figure 100).

Other manifestations of disseminated gonococcal infection are hepatitis, endocarditis and meningitis. Diagnosis of uncomplicated gonorrhea in males can be made by Gram staining of the urethral discharge with demonstration of Gram-negative intracellular diplococci (see Figure 2), whereas culture is required in females.

A sexually active girl (Figure 101) presented with fever, chills and arthralgia, and several papular lesions over the face and extremities.

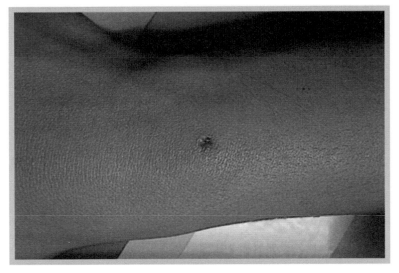

Figure 101

Cultures of blood, cervix and skin pustules were negative for *N. gonorrhoeae*. However, punch biopsy of a pustule was positive for diplococci on immunofluorescent analysis. Parenteral ceftriaxone therapy effected prompt recovery.

Genital herpes simplex

Most cases of genital herpes (herpetic vulvovaginitis and herpes progenitalis) are caused by HSV serotype 2 (HSV-2). Infection is usually asymptomatic, although HSV is recognized to be the most common etiology of genital ulcers. Lesions are painful.

A typical herpes progenitalis penile ulcer in a teenager may heal spontaneously without antiviral therapy. HSV-2 vulvitis (Figure 102) and cervicitis with perineal dermatitis were diagnosed in an adolescent. A smear of the cervical vesicles (Tzanck preparation) revealed multinucleated giant cells with intracytoplasmic inclusions and eosinophilic intranuclear inclusions (Pananicolaou stain).

97

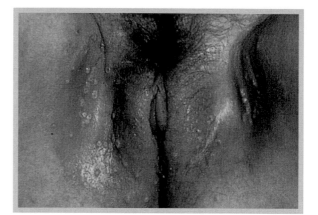

Figure 102

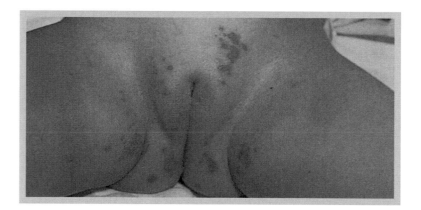

Figure 103

Infection may also occur in young children, transmitted from the contaminated hands of care-givers. The infant shown in Figure 103 has HSV-2 diaper dermatitis that resolved spontaneously in 12 days without sequelae.

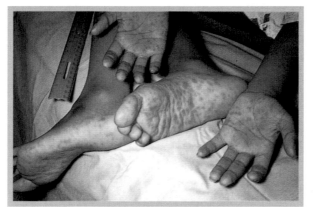

Figure 104

Syphilis

Syphilis caused by the *T. pallidum* spirochete has continued to be a hidden epidemic among adolescents and young adults. Asymptomatic disease is twice as common in 15–19-year-old females as in males in this age group.

There are three clinical stages: primary, with mucocutaneous (genital, anal, oral) painless ulcers; secondary, with a maculopapular exanthem involving the palms and soles, and generalized lymphadenopathy, fever, malaise, arthralgia, splenomegaly and genital or perianal condylomata lata; and teriary or latent (from more than 6 months to more than 2 years), with neurosyphilis and/or rarely cardiovascular or gummatous disease. Moth-eaten alopecia may be seen in the secondary stage. Diagnostic tests include screening non-treponemal (VDRL, RPR, ART) and specific treponemal (FTA-ABS, MHA-TP) tests.

Secondary syphilitic copper-colored papulosquamous rash lasting 1 week was seen on the palms and soles of the girl shown in Figure 104 following sexual abuse. Examination revealed a vaginal chancre containing numerous *T. pallidum* organisms on dark-field

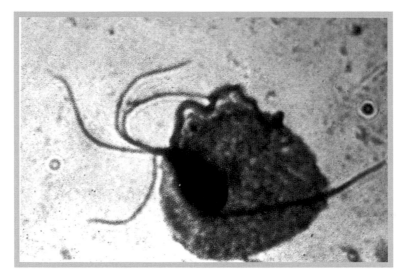

Figure 105

examination. A VDRL test was positive and penicillin therapy proved effective.

Trichomoniasis

Trichomonas vaginalis is a flagellated protozoan (Figure 105) whose presence is often asymptomatic in females. Moderate to heavy colonization produces a yellow–green discharge with a pH > 4.5 and a fishy odor associated with pruritic vaginitis, cervicitis or urethritis. Infection in postmenarchal girls strongly suggests sexual activity whereas, in premenarchal children, trichomoniasis necessitates careful examination for sexual abuse.

Diagnosis is made by direct microscopic examination (wet preparation) of fresh vaginal discharge. Males are more frequently symptomatic, with urethritis or prostatitis.

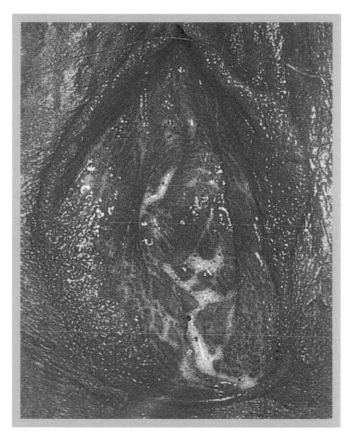

Figure 106

Vaginosis

Bacterial vaginosis, also called non-specific vaginitis, results from the overgrowth of *Gardnerella vaginalis* and/or anaerobes such as *Mobiluncus* species. The diagnosis is suggested by the presence of a homogeneous discharge (Figure 106) with a pH > 4.5 and a positive amine odor test. More specific is the presence of clue cells (Figure 107), epithelial cells containing clumps of bacteria on their surface.

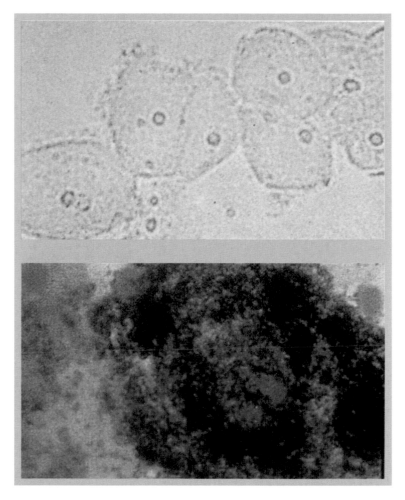

Figure 107

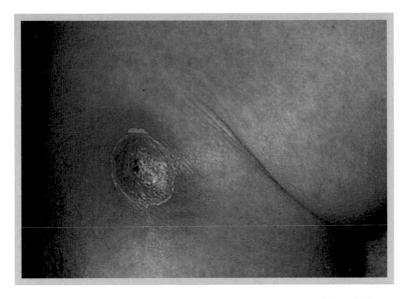

Figure 108

Skin, soft tissue and lymph node infections

Abscesses

Boils or furuncles (Figure 108) are the major manifestation of *S. aureus* infections when they occur in the skin. Multiloculated furuncles are called carbuncles. Group A β-hemolytic streptococci are often associated with abscesses in the head and neck areas, and Gram-negative enteric bacilli are implicated as the cause of abscesses on the abdomen and pelvis, particularly on perianal and perirectal areas.

Actinomycosis

The four most common clinical presentations of infection with *Actinomyces israelii* are cervicofacial ('lumpy-bumpy jaw'; Figure 109), abdominal, thoracic/mediastinal and pelvic. Pathogenesis is presumed to begin with mucous membrane trauma in patients with poor oral

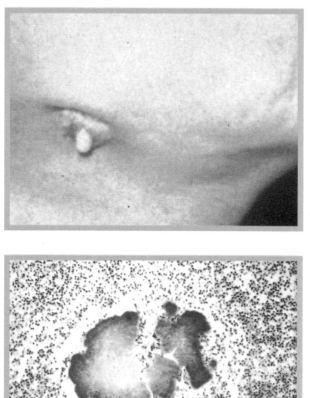

Figure 109

Figure 110

hygiene, aspiration into the lung of endogenous flora of the oral cavity or perforation of an abdominal hollow viscus such as a ruptured appendix.

Pelvic disease is usually associated with the presence of an intrauterine device. The disease is chronic, with sites of infection containing polymorphonuclear leukocytes and monocytes/macrophages together with characteristic sulfur granules (Figure 110). Material for

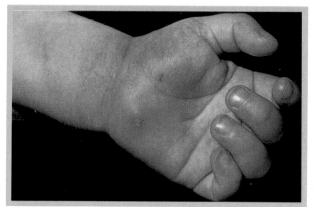

Figure 111

microscopic examination is best obtained from purulent sinus tract drainage. Pulmonary actinomycosis may dissect into the mediastinum to produce an abscess with involvement of the adjacent ribs.

Animal bites

Punctures are more likely to become infected than tears or open lacerations. As most cat bites result in punctures, they have a high rate of infection (30–50%), whereas dog bites, which usually result in tears or lacerations, have low infection rates (6–10%).

Infections following both cat and dog bites are usually due to *Pasteurella multocida*, although *Staphylococcus aureus* and *S. intermedius* are also frequent pathogens. Infection with *P. multocida* is apparent as early as 12 h after a bite, with swelling, redness and tenderness around the puncture marks (Figure 111, a cat bite).

Staining of purulent discharge from these lesions may reveal Gram-negative bacilli. Dog bites, and rarely cat bites, may become infected with *Capnocytophaga canimorsus*, which is associated with a high incidence of septicemia and death in asplenic and immuno-compromised patients.

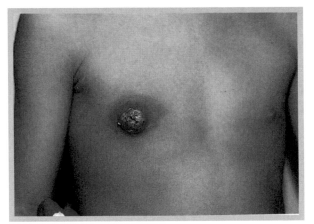

Figure 112

Breast abscess

Coagulase-positive staphylococci account for 90% of breast abscesses. The majority are seen in neonates during the first 2 weeks of life in association with physiological breast enlargement, but infection may occur at any age in girls. As with other staphylococcal soft-tissue infections, the prominent feature is abscess formation with a minimal surrounding cellulitis (Figure 112). Fever and constitutional symptoms are rarely present.

Surgical drainage is required for cure as inadequate treatment may result in destruction of the breast bud and cosmetically unacceptable reduction in ultimate breast size. In this case (Figure 113), the breast bud was identified and preserved during surgery while the abscess was drained.

Cat-scratch disease

Bartonella henselae is the cause of cat-scratch disease (CSD), which usually presents with chronic adenopathy or chronic lymphadenitis (Figure 114) more than 3 weeks following exposure to kittens. This boy had a fever of up to 104°F, with a headache, anorexia, fatigue,

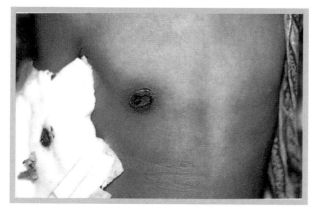

Figure 113

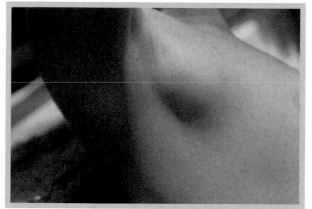

Figure 114

tender axillary lymphadenitis and a weight loss over 7–10 days of 9 lb (4.08 kg). He had allowed a kitten to sleep in bed with him and thus received multiple scratches. A crusted primary inoculation papule on his upper chest was noted 4 weeks prior to his illness. A CSD skin test produced a 30-mm area of induration. The adenitis resolved spontaneously within 4 months.

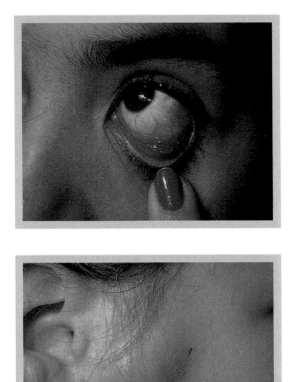

Figure 115

Figure 116

CSD is the most common cause of Parinaud's oculoglandular syndrome, a combination of conjunctivitis and preauricular adenitis. The child shown in Figure 115 suffered a corneal abrasion while playing with a cat. The injury produced a conjunctival granuloma persisting 3–4 weeks. Parotid gland swelling (Figure 116) due to intra-parotid adenopathy was present for 2–3 months.

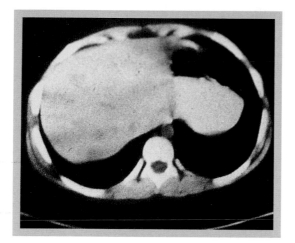

Figure 117

CSD can also cause multifocal hepatosplenic abscesses and encephalitis. A child had high fever for 16 days, anorexia and lethargy, with cervical adenopathy and splenomegaly. Multiple kitten scratches produced papules on both arms that appeared 2 weeks prior to the illness. The family cat had five kittens that were heavily flea-infested.

Ultrasonography and CT revealed multiple hypoechoic defects in the liver and spleen (Figure 117). The erythrocyte sedimentation rate was 90 mm/h. An indirect fluorescent antibody titer for B. henselae was 1 : 8193; a CSD skin test resulted in a 22-mm area of induration.

Five days after ciprofloxacin treatment began, the patient was admitted to hospital with recurrent grand mal seizures and fever. Recovery was rapid with a normal neurological examination 7 days later. Repeat ultrasound scans of the liver and spleen were normal.

A gallium scan of a similar patient showed multiple areas of increased uptake in the liver (Figure 118). Liver biopsy revealed a granuloma containing CSD bacilli, identified with a Warthin–Starry silver stain (Figure 119).

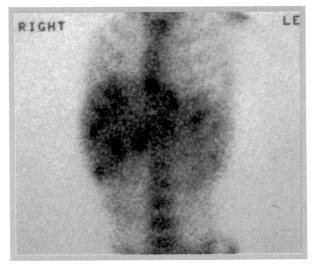

Figure 118

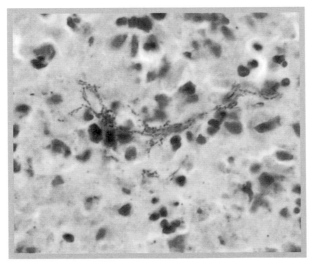

Figure 119

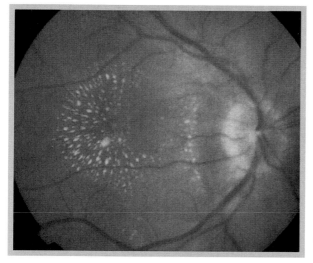

Figure 120

A young man had flu-like symptoms for 3 weeks prior to experiencing decreased vision in his right eye. A papular rash was noted on his abdomen and arms which was attributed to flea bites and cat scratches. Other findings were submental adenopathy and splenomegaly.

Examination of the right fundus revealed papilledema with a macular star and retinal white spots (Figure 120). Visual acuity was 20/50. The left fundus was normal. A CSD skin test resulting in a 35-mm area of induration confirmed the diagnosis. Spontaneous resolution of adenopathy and return of normal vision occurred in 3 months, and the maculopapular rash resolved in 6 months.

Cellulitis

Infection of the skin and subcutaneous tissue is manifest by spreading erythema and edema with a well-defined margin, usually from a point source, frequently an abrasion, insect bites or an infected varicella lesion. Group A β-hemolytic streptococci are the likely pathogens, especially when the cellulitis appears to originate from a point source on the skin.

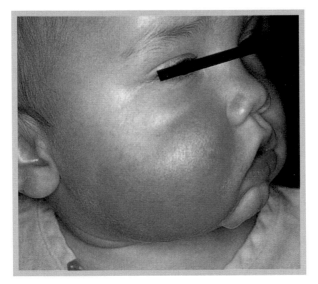

Figure 121

Buccal cellulitis due to *Haemophilus influenzae* type b, or Hib (Figure 121), was a well-recognized form of cellulitis before the routine administration of Hib conjugate vaccines. Hib cellulitis occurs primarily in infants and young children, most of whom are febrile and bacteremic. The cellulitis arises in areas with intact overlying skin, presumably as a result of the bacteremia.

At present, *Streptococcus pneumoniae* is the most common etiology of periorbital (preseptal) cellulitis that occurs as an extension of sinus infection (Figure 122). CT of the orbits shows a diffuse swelling in the preseptal area with normal retro-orbital anatomy (Figure 123).

In contrast, the child shown in Figure 124 with orbital or postseptal cellulitis had Hib bacteremia. CT of the orbit (Figure 125) shows opacification of the right ethmoid sinuses with subperiosteal abscess formation in the right retro-orbital space, and displacement of the eye and orbit contents forwards to produce proptosis.

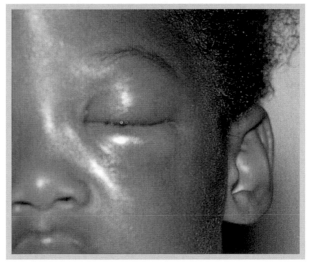

Figure 122

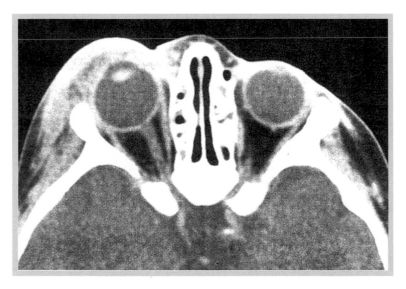

Figure 123

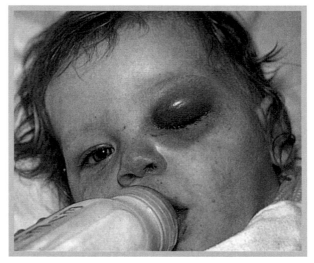

Figure 124

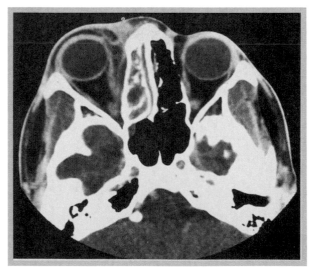

Figure 125

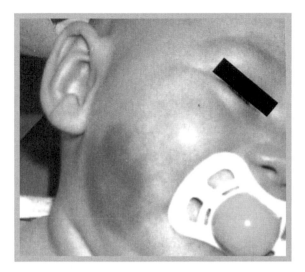

Figure 126

Erysipelas

This is superficial cellulitis of the skin with marked lymphatic vessel involvement caused by group A β-hemolytic streptococci (GABHS). The face and scalp are most often infected following a break in the skin. A small area of redness gradually enlarges into a hot, painful, shiny bright red, well-demarcated plaque with surrounding edema and induration.

While recovering from chickenpox, a boy developed acutely tender, red, swollen skin over both cheeks and the nasal bridge after having scratched his left upper eyelid. Three days later, there was facial edema, fever to 106°F and irritability. The patient experienced a generalized seizure 1 day prior to admission. Culture of the eye exudate produced a heavy growth of GABHS. Oxacillin therapy was effective with recovery in 48 h. Cultures of pustules on the mother's finger also grew GABHS.

The infant shown in Figure 126 had erysipelas which was associated with otitis media and GABHS bacteremia.

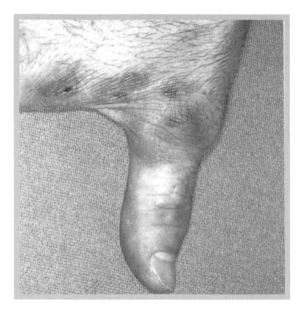

Figure 127

Erysipeloid

The teenager in Figure 127 was injured by a catfish spike while cleaning the fish. A localized painful cellulitis was noted 2 days later. *Erysipelothrix rhusiopathiae* was cultured from a soft-tissue biopsy. This organism is a commensal colonizing bacteria of many animal species, which renders contact with wild game or foodstuffs the usual risk factor to humans.

Absence of suppuration is characteristic, in contrast to infection due to staphylococci. Infection may also result in chronic dermatitis and disseminate to cause sepsis or endocarditis. Untreated local infection will usually abate within 3 weeks, whereas therapy with oral penicillin produces a much more rapid resolution.

Erythema nodosum

These red tender nodular lesions, usually on the pretibial surface of the legs, represent a delayed hypersensitivity skin reaction. The most

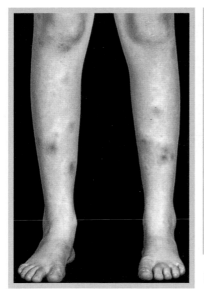

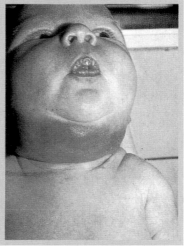

Figure 129

Figure 128

common precipitating factor is medication, in particular, contraceptive pills taken by adolescents. However, infectious diseases are also often incriminated, particularly GABHS, tuberculosis, sarcoidosis, cat-scratch disease and coccidioidomycosis (Figure 128).

The nodular lesions of erythema nodosum have indistinct borders and persist for 2–6 weeks.

Ludwig's angina

An extensive, rapidly progressive cellulitis of the floor of the mouth may result in sepsis and/or airway obstruction (Figure 129). The causative pathogens, in order of frequency, are *Staphylococcus aureus*, *Streptococcus pneumoniae*, *Haemophilus influenzae*, *Escherichia coli*, *Pseudomonas* species, *Moraxella catarrhalis*, fusiform bacilli and anaerobic streptococci.

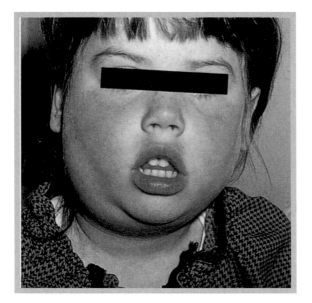

Figure 130

Treatment includes maintenance of the airway, usually with endotracheal intubation, intravenous antibiotics and surgical drainage if fluctuation is present.

Mumps

Parotitis is rarely seen in developed countries, a result of the routine administration of measles–mumps–rubella (MMR) vaccine, which began in the early 1970s.

Mumps is characterized by gradual enlargement of one parotid gland over the course of 1–3 days (Figure 130). This may be followed by involvement of the opposite parotid gland in 25–35% of cases and often the submaxillary glands on the affected sides as well. Swelling of either or both parotid glands increases for several days. Although there is only mild tenderness on palpation, there may be intense parotid pain with chewing. Fever is low grade (< 102°F). Parotid swelling begins to subside after several days and resolves after 2–3 weeks. In an

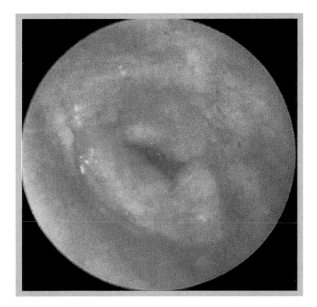

Figure 131

estimated 50% of infections, mumps is so mild as to remain undiagnosed.

Otitis externa

Retention of water within the ear may result in bacterial replication and inflammation of the external ear canal (Figure 131). Recovered pathogens are those that commonly colonize the skin and thrive in moist environments, such as *Pseudomonas aeruginosa*, *Staphylococcus aureus*, *Proteus vulgaris* and Enterobacteriaceae.

Therapy of otitis externa is directed at eradication of probable organisms with broad-spectrum antibiotics, which can be accomplished with a brief 5–7-day course. Children who swim frequently or have had repeated bouts of otitis externa should instill an acidified alcohol solution into the external canals after swimming or showering.

A serious form of this infection, caused by *P. aeruginosa* (Figure 132), is seen in insulin-dependent diabetes and patients with immuno-

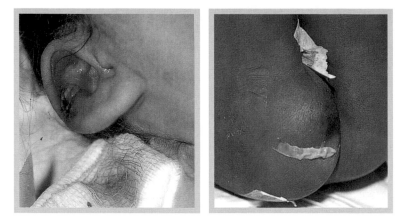

Figure 132   Figure 133

deficiency. The organism has a unique propensity for cartilage and may rapidly extend into deeper structures.

Perianal abscess

Abscesses in the perianal region (Figure 133) are almost always associated with anaerobic bacteria, although mixed infection with *Staphylococcus aureus*, *Escherichia coli*, streptococci and other coliforms is common. As with all cutaneous abscesses, incision with drainage is the most important aspect of therapy. In contrast to infection in other anatomical areas, simple drainage may be inadequate. Fistulae must be identified, opened and excised. Perianal (perirectal) abscesses therefore require surgical consultation. Antimicrobial therapy is only necessary for extensive cellulitis, systemic symptoms or an immuno-compromised host.

Pityriasis alba

This common skin disorder of unknown etiology is characterized by the appearance of one or more hypopigmented patches on the face (usually the cheek; Figure 134), neck and upper trunk. The patches measure from one to several centimeters in diameter and have distinct

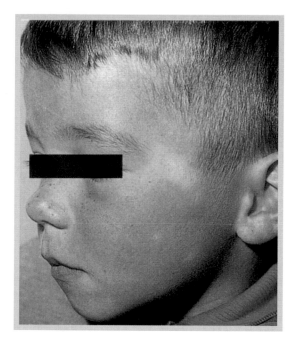

Figure 134

margins; there may be fine brawny scales. The lesions are more prominent in darker-skinned subjects with recent sun exposure and tanning of the adjacent skin. The rash resolves spontaneously within several weeks.

Pityriasis rosea

The characteristic skin eruption of pityriasis rosea usually permits early clinical diagnosis. The disease is seen in school-age children and adolescents, and begins with a single skin lesion, the 'herald patch' (Figure 135). This single, round or oval, reddish-brown lesion appears on the trunk or proximal extremities, where it may resemble tinea corporis. The patch is one to several centimeters in diameter with fine scaling and elevation of the outer border, and appears several days before the generalized eruption.

121

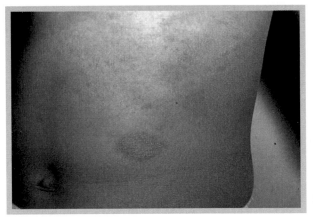

Figure 135

Although individual skin lesions in the later rash are similar to the herald patch, such lesions are smaller, measuring from only a few millimeters to 1–3 cm in diameter, pink and oval-shaped. They may appear in one or several crops and persist for 2–12 weeks. The long axis of each plaque is usually aligned parallel to cutaneous lines of cleavage so that the overall configuration of lesions on the back resembles a Christmas tree. Most of these oval plaques have slightly raised edges with central clearing and a fine collarette of scales attached at the inner edge of the border (Figure 136). Mild pruritus is the only other manifestation. The cause of pityriasis rosea is unknown, but presumed to be of viral etiology.

Pyoderma

In pediatric patients, pyoderma refers to superficial purulent skin infections in early infancy, primarily staphylococcal disease in the newborn, which occurs in two clinical forms – pustular and bullous. The pustular form presents with a few to many skin pustules, primarily over the diaper area and trunk. This neonatal pyoderma is highly associated with infection due to phage group I, type 80/81 *Staphylococcus aureus*, strains that were most prevalent prior to 1970. These organisms are highly virulent, and often associated with invasive and life-threatening disease.

Figure 136

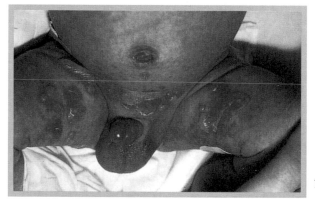

Figure 137

However, these strains have been largely replaced by exfoliatin toxin-producing strains, commonly phage group II, type 71 S. aureus. Although these strains are less invasive, superficial infections in newborns, who do not yet have passive immunity to their exfoliatin toxins, results in generalized erythroderma and desquamation or Ritter's disease. Superficial infection with these strains in newborns without passive antibodies to exfoliatin toxins results in bullous pyoderma (Figure 137).

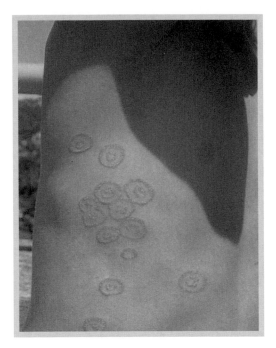

Figure 138

Ringworm

Tinea corporis is an infection caused by a number of fungi (dermatophytes) that may infect the stratum corneum of glabrous skin. These
infections take the form of circular lesions with expanding outer
borders, often with central clearing as the infection spreads (Figure
138). The outer edge of the lesion usually has a raised border with
minute vesicles and scales. At present, the most common cause of
ringworm in the USA and Europe is any of several species of
Trichophyton including *T. tonsurans*, *T. mentagrophytes* and *T. rubrum*.

Ringworm of the scalp (tinea capitis) is manifested by circular patches
of hair loss which, on close inspection, reveal individual hairs that are
broken off at different levels above the scalp. There may be an intense
and severe inflammatory reaction with marked boggy swelling of the
area, vesicle and pustule formation, crateriform lesions from which pus

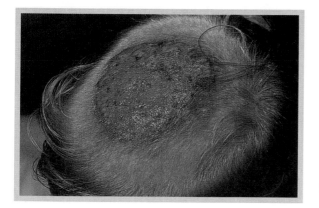

Figure 139

may exude, often matting the hair in a purulent crust called a kerion (Figure 139).

Other forms of skin infection due to dermatophytes that may not produce typical ringworm lesions include tinea pedis or 'athlete's foot', caused by *T. rubrum* and *Epidermophyton floccosum* (Figure 140) and *E. floccosum* infection of the groin, resulting in tinea cruris or 'jock itch' (Figure 141).

Scrofula

Although pulmonary disease is the most frequent form of tuberculosis, extrapulmonary disease following hematogenous dissemination is seen within 1 year of initial lung infection in about 25% of children less than 5 years old, as well as in immunosuppressed adults. Cervical lymphadenitis, termed scrofula, is the most common manifestation of disseminated tuberculosis.

A boy developed femoral lymphadenitis with serosanguineous discharge of 4 months' duration from which *Mycobacterium tuberculosis* was recovered. His chest X-ray was normal, but the intradermal purified protein derivative (IPPD) tuberculin skin test produced a 28-mm area of induration. Biopsy of the mass revealed caseating necrosis, and acid-fast bacilli were identified in gastric aspirates. Both nodes resolved in 5 months after treatment with isoniazid and rifampin.

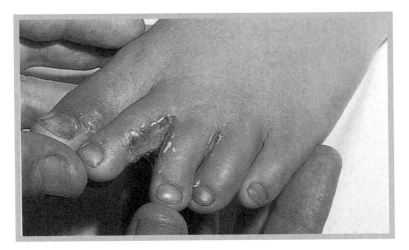

Figure 140

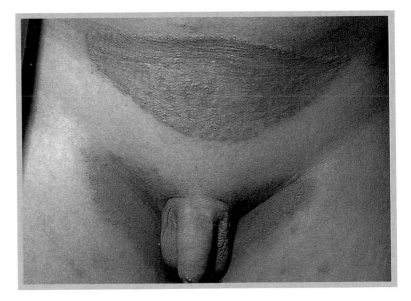

Figure 141

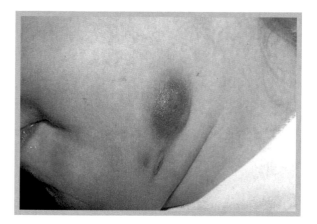

Figure 142

Non-tuberculous mycobacteria are also known to cause scrofula (Figure 142). This healthy child had a tender parotid abscess and right submandibular adenitis for 5 weeks. Biopsy of the node revealed caseating necrosis and a culture grew M. *scrofulaceum* on Lowenstein–Jensen medium. A Mantoux tuberculin skin test resulted in only 6 mm of induration.

Isoniazid and rifampin were ineffective. Spontaneous discharge of caseous matter over several weeks was followed by incomplete healing after 6 months. Excisional surgery is the ideal therapy for non-tuberculous mycobacterial adenopathy.

Sporotrichosis

Sporothrix schenckii, a dimorphous fungus commonly isolated from soil and plants, may produce skin and subcutaneous disease in the normal host and disseminated infection in immunocompromised patients. Infection occurs in all age groups, but is most common in adult males who are likely to be exposed to contaminated soil or vegetation.

Lymphocutaneous sporotrichosis is the most common manifestation of the disease, seen in 75% of all cases. Infection follows a wound from a splinter, thorn, glass, cat bite or cat scratch contaminated with the organism.

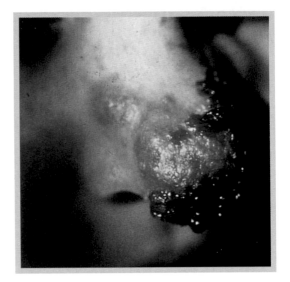

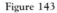
Figure 143

The initial lesion is characterized by a small firm, painless dusky-colored papule that develops at the site of trauma 1–12 weeks after inoculation, then slowly enlarges to eventually ulcerate. In children, lesions on the face and trunk are fairly common.

The child shown in Figure 143 has an infection on the nose. Localized forms of the disorder range from scaly maculopapular lesions to verrucous and weeping ulcerations with or without satellite lesions. Itraconazole is now the treatment of choice for cutaneous sporotrichosis.

Swimming pool, fish tank or Chesapeake Bay granuloma

Mycobacterium marinum is an acid-fast organism related to M. *tuberculosis* that produces chronic cutaneous lesions following injury during exposure to contaminated water. A child presented with a 3.5-month history of granuloma on his foot (Figure 144) which slowly developed after scraping his foot on a barnacle in Chesapeake Bay.

A tuberculin skin test (IPPD) produced a 13-mm area of induration. Skin excisional biopsy showed non-caseating granuloma. Culture was

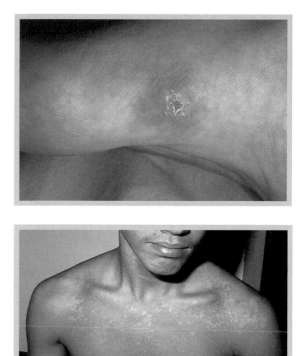

Figure 144

Figure 145

positive for M. *marinum*. Recovery was prompt, with no recurrence after 5 years.

Tinea versicolor

This infection of the striatum corneum of the skin is caused by the dimorphic yeast *Malassezia furfur*. Round or oval hypopigmented or, less commonly, hyperpigmented lesions varying from a few millimeters to 2–3 cm in diameter occur most usually on the neck and shoulders (Figure 145). Wet-mount potassium hydroxide preparations of skin

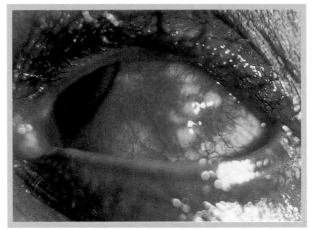

Figure 146

scrapings from these lesions reveal hyphae and clusters of spores in a pattern often referred to as 'spaghetti and meatballs'.

Tularemia

There are six classical forms of the tick-transmitted disease caused by *Francisella tularensis*: ulceroglandular, glandular, oculoglandular, also called Parinaud oculoglandular syndrome (Figure 146), oropharyngeal typhoidal, and pneumonic. Pulmonary involvement is much less common in children than in adults. Regardless of disease form, the incubation period is 3–4 days; general symptoms are abrupt, consisting of fever, chills, headache and myalgia.

Treated or untreated, adenitis often progresses, thus requiring drainage for relief of symptoms (Figure 147). This needs to be carried out with caution in patients who have not completed therapy, as the exudates may be infectious. Similarly, aspirated exudates should not be cultured because of risk to laboratory personnel.

Serological agglutination tests, the usual diagnostic method, are not positive until the second or third week of illness. Therefore, empirical

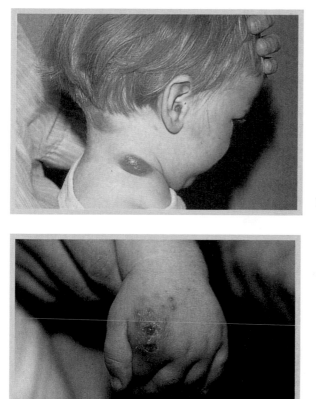

Figure 147

Figure 148

therapy must be considered for patients with high fever and adenitis following tick exposure in endemic regions, particularly during compatible seasons.

Disease is occasionally transmitted from the bite of an infected animal, as was the case in the child bitten by a pet squirrel (Figure 148). Three days following the bite, she developed cellulitis and painful axillary adenitis.

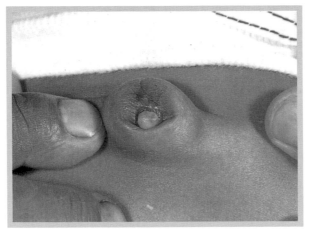

Figure 149

Umbilical granuloma

Pyogenic granuloma at the base of the umbilicus are commonly seen in neonates during the first few weeks of life. The lesions are round or oval, reddish-brown, smooth, firm and moist, varying in diameter from 2–3 mm to 1.0 cm or more (Figure 149). They are often pedunculated and tend to bleed with minor trauma. Histologically, they are composed of granulomatous tissue with neovascular proliferation.

Warts (verrucae)

Human papillomavirus (HPV)-induced intraepidermal tumors are some of the most common skin disorders seen in patients of all ages. There are four basic forms of verrucae caused by different types of HPV: verruca vulgaris (HPV types 1, 2, 4 or 7), verruca plana (HPV 3, 10, or 26), verruca plantaris, and condylomata acuminata (HPV 6, 11, 16 or 18).

The common wart appears as a single or multiple papules with an irregular rough surface (Figure 150) or, in areas of trauma, as linear warts, termed the Koebner phenomenon (Figure 151). Lesions are usually on the extremities, but may involve other areas of the skin, including the scalp and genitalia.

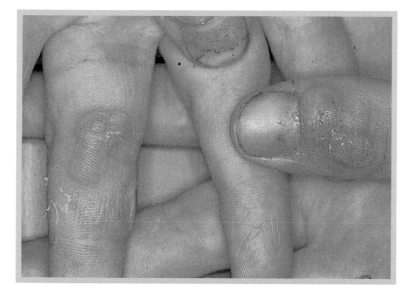

Figure 150

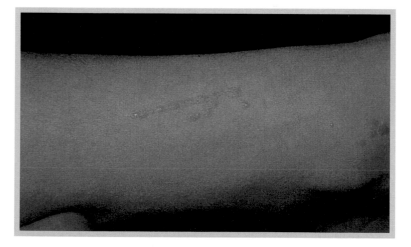

Figure 151

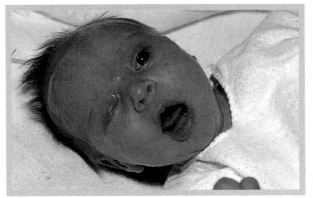

Figure 152

Infections specific to organ systems

Bell palsy

Also known as facial nerve paralysis, the condition is peripheral in origin. Occasionally, it is secondary to otitis media, presumably as a result of extension of inflammation to cranial nerve VII as it courses through the bony canal.

The infant in Figure 152 has otitis media in the left ear and a left facial paralysis, identified by the inability to draw his mouth downwards while crying and to fully close his left eye. Paralysis may also follow viral infection, with a maculopapular rash, left facial nerve involvement, and a positive stool and throat culture for echovirus 9. Recent studies have documented the presence of herpes simplex virus, using polymerase chain reaction (PCR), in a high percentage of facial nerve biopsies of Bell palsy patients.

Brain abscess

Localized suppurative infection of the brain usually occurs by direct extension from sinus or mastoid disease. Historically, it was more commonly a sequela of bacterial meningitis but, nowadays, only meningitis caused by *Citrobacter diversus* in neonates commonly produces intracerebral abscesses. Other predisposing factors are congenital heart disease with right-to-left shunts and head trauma.

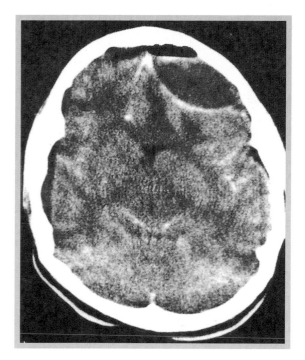

Figure 153

Clinical manifestations may be subtle, with fever, headache and vomiting being the most common. At present, CT is the procedure of choice for demonstrating abscesses, as in the preoperative CT study shown in Figure 153, which shows a large right frontal abscess associated with maxillary and ethmoid sinus infection.

Meningoencephalitis

The majority of viral and postviral neurological diseases are benign and self-limiting, with enteroviruses causing more than 80% of cases in children. Some viral neurological diseases are more severe, in particular, herpes encephalitis, some equine encephalitides, and Guillain–Barré and Reye syndromes.

Several viruses that cause meningoencephalitis appear to be clinically similar. Seasonal occurrence and associated systemic signs and

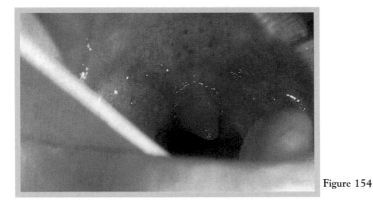

Figure 154

symptoms may suggest a specific viral cause. Equine encephalitis, a mosquito-borne viral disease, typically occurs during the warmer months, whereas herpes encephalitis is sporadic.

A boy developed persistent coryza, lethargy, headache, fever, irritability and anorexia of 3–4 days' duration. A maculopapular rash with truncal and oropharyngeal petechiae was accompanied by nuchal rigidity. Buccal pseudo-Koplik papules (Figure 154) were also observed. Echovirus 9 was isolated from pharyngeal washings.

Herpes encephalitis beyond the neonatal period usually occurs in the absence of cutaneous or other focal manifestations. Patients present with signs and symptoms of severe encephalitis such as high fever, changes in mental status, seizures and focal neurological findings.

CSF examination classically yields an increase in mononuclear leukocytes and red blood cells. However, as less than 5% of cases have positive CSF cultures, brain biopsy for histological examination and culture is the best method for confirming the diagnosis. The site of biopsy may be determined by MRI. The brain biopsy in Figure 155 shows scattered areas of cells containing cytoplasmic viral inclusions indicative of herpes simplex infection.

Varicella–zoster virus has never been isolated from the CSF of an immune-competent host with encephalitis, but may be cultured from

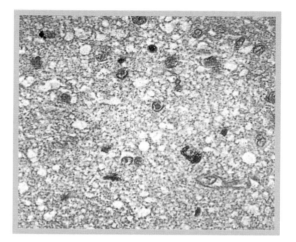

Figure 155

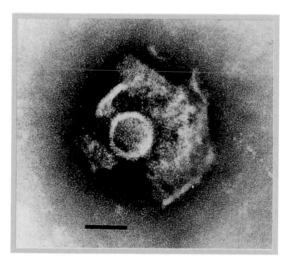

Figure 156

the CSF of immunosuppressed patients or identified by electron microscopy, as seen in this child (Figure 156) receiving immuno-suppressive chemotherapy for leukemia who developed chickenpox and encephalitis.

Croup

Laryngotracheobronchitis (LTB) is the most common cause of acute partial upper airway obstruction in children. The terminology used to describe this disease and its differential diagnosis have been confusing. Laryngotracheobronchitis refers to partial airway obstruction caused by a viral infection, with erythema and edema concentrated mostly in the subglottic area. The organism responsible is usually a parainfluenza virus (types 1, 2 or 3), although other organisms may cause epidemic Laryngotracheobronchitis (respiratory syncytial virus, influenza virus and rhinovirus).

The term croup is used to describe obstruction usually due to infection but, occasionally, by a foreign body or other etiology. Croup is characterized by a persistent resonant barking cough, hoarseness and stridor.

Lateral neck radiography may be helpful in differentiating the cause, whether viral, foreign body, retropharyngeal abscess or bacterial epiglottitis. These studies should be taken with the neck extended in the 'sniffing dog' position to allow optimal visualization of the trachea, larynx and supralaryngeal structures.

The normal lateral radiograph in Figure 157 shows the tracheal air column becoming wider and more radiolucent in the larynx. The epiglottis has the configuration of the tip of a little-finger on lateral projection, the so-called little finger sign, and the arytenoid folds are poorly visualized. The airway is patent through these structures.

In a lateral neck radiograph of a child with subglottic viral croup (Figure 158), the tracheal air column becomes narrow and less radiolucent in the larynx due to laryngeal edema, but the epiglottis is normal.

Pertussis

Whooping cough is a communicable infection of the respiratory tract characterized by repeated paroxysms of coughing. Young infants with severe disease may have numerous paroxysms terminating in cyanosis and apnea. Such episodes may be fatal if resuscitation is not provided.

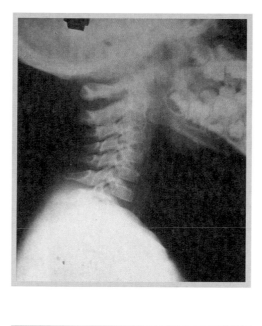

Figure 157

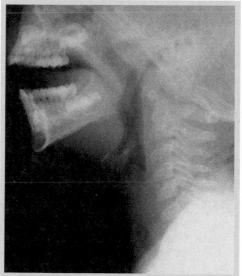

Figure 158

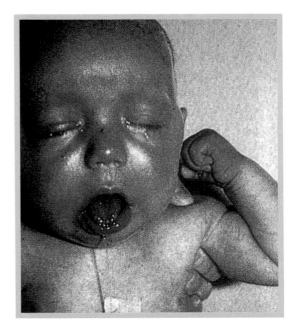

Figure 159

The infant in Figure 159 shows developing cyanosis with accumulation of thick ropy airway secretions during a severe coughing paroxysm. The face of a child with pertussis, who had numerous bouts of severe coughing paroxysms daily, showed the resultant edema of the eyelids and scleral hemorrhage.

Pneumonia

Approximately 50% of pediatric pneumonias are caused by viral agents alone. Of these, 50% are attributed to respiratory syncytial virus (RSV) and 25% to parainfluenza virus types 1 and 3. A smaller number of cases are due to influenza A and B, adenovirus or rhinovirus. Three of these subgroups (RSV, parainfluenza virus and influenza virus) are seen almost exclusively during the winter months. Adenovirus is the common viral pathogen during the remainder of the year.

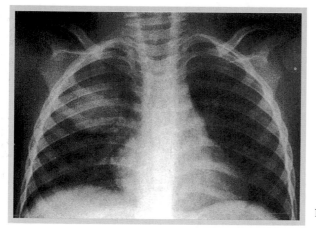

Figure 160

Such seasonal clustering of viral pneumonias suggests an increased likelihood of bacterial causes during the spring, summer and fall. Determination of the bacterial organisms causing pneumonia is primarily related to the age of the pediatric patient. Other data used to identify probable cause include associated clinical signs and symptoms, chest X-ray findings and diagnostic laboratory tests.

A 1-year-old presented with fever, cough, dyspnea, anorexia and irritability over 24 h. Examination revealed an acutely ill infant with tachypnea and tachycardia. Tabular breathing with dullness on percussion was noted over the right superior anterolateral chest. The white cell count was 22 000/mm³ with 75% polymorphonuclear leukocytes and 10% band forms. Chest X-ray revealed a right upper anterior lobe pneumonia (Figure 160). Blood culture grew *Klebsiella pneumoniae*. Intramuscular ampicillin for 36 h was ineffective, whereas intramuscular kanamycin produced an excellent response, with complete recovery 10 days after starting treatment.

Tracheal obstruction due to a mediastinal mass occurred in a 2-year-old who was hospitalized with sudden onset of stridor, dyspnea, tachypnea and fever. She had a history of persistent brassy cough and mild stridor for 5–6 weeks. The healthy mother and two siblings were

141

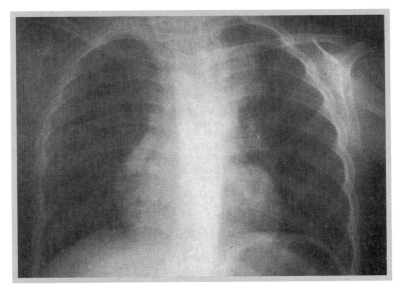

Figure 161

tuberculin skin test-negative. The father was an expatriot of Nigeria whose health was unknown.

Chest X-ray revealed clear lung fields, but marked superior mediastinal fullness (Figure 161). CT revealed a mass compressing the trachea. A tuberculin skin test was positive with a 32-mm area of induration. Following endotracheal intubation, a thoracotomy revealed a 5 x 4 x 3 cm mass of matted lymph nodes. Histological examination of an excisional biopsy showed multiple caseating granulomas containing acid-fast bacilli. *Mycobacterium tuberculosis* was cultured and was found to be susceptible to all anti-tuberculous drugs.

There was a minimal response after 18 days of treatment with intramuscular isoniazid, rifampin and streptomycin. Prednisone and dexamethasome therapy were effective, resulting in normal respiratory efforts after 5 days. Recovery was complete in 3 months, but chest X-ray showed persistent hilar adenopathy for 5 months.

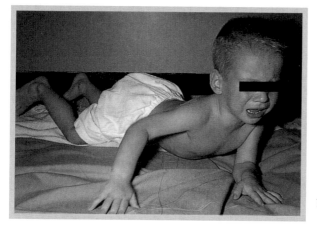

Figure 162

Discitis

This benign, usually self-limiting, inflammatory process or infection of the intervertebral disc space and vertebral endplate mostly affects children less than 5 years of age. Responsible pathogens most commonly are *Staphylococcus aureus* or *S. epidermidis*, although cultures of the disc space are positive in less than 50% of cases. Clinical manifestations include irritability, limp, refusal to sit, stand or walk and resistance to being moved.

Examination is normal except for an immobile irritable child with diffuse spinal tenderness and/or paraspinal muscle spasm. The white cell count is usually normal, but the erythrocyte sedimentation rate is often elevated. Radiography of the lumbar spine is normal during the first 2–3 weeks. However, a technetium bone scan, CT or MRI will reveal early intervertebral involvement.

Treatment consists of analgesics; immobilization of the spine is helpful and, in selected cases, antistaphylococcal antibiotics. The prognosis is excellent.

The child in Figure 162 developed severe back pain with spinal rigidity gradually over 3–4 weeks. He was afebrile and comfortable

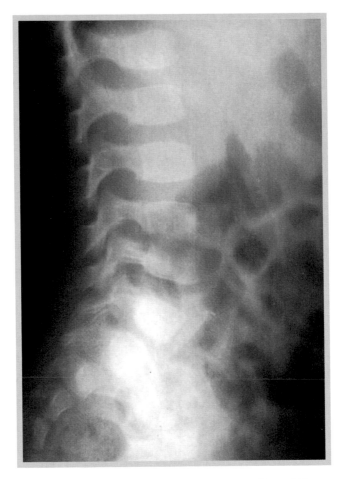

Figure 163

except when moved. There was marked spasm of the paraspinal muscles and a positive Gowers' sign. Radiography revealed narrowing of the L3/L4 disc space, with irregularity of the adjacent vertebral body endplates (Figure 163).

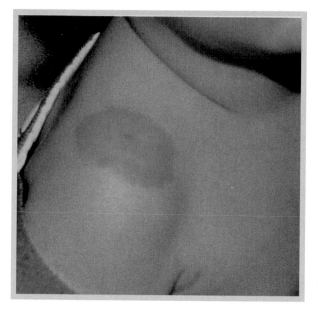

Figure 164

Lyme disease

Infection caused by *Borrelia burgdorferi* begins with a characteristic rash, erythema migrans (Figure 164), at the site of a tick bite. Documentation of this rash remains the best diagnostic method, as all current laboratory assays are notoriously non-specific.

By definition, the lesions are more than 5 cm in diameter, often with central clearing. If untreated during the next several weeks, patients may develop multiple similar skin lesions with periorbital edema, conjunctivitis, fever and arthralgia. Late manifestations include arthritis, carditis, facial nerve (Bell) palsy and peripheral radiculo-neuropathy.

Endemic regions in the USA are the Northeast, Midwest and California, which correlate with the distribution of the tick vectors, *Ixodes scapularis* and *I. pacificus*.

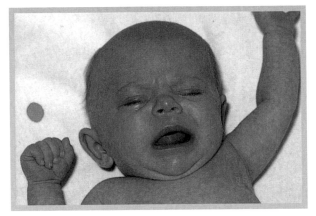

Figure 165

Mastoiditis

This refers to infection of the posterior process of the temporal bone, almost exclusively as a consequence of prolonged middle ear suppuration. Disease may evolve with either acute or chronic manifestations; these two presentations are distinctly different in bacterial etiology and management requirements.

The characteristic presentation is an irritable child with high fever, and retroauricular swelling and erythema that either tilts the pinna outwards and downwards or elevates the earlobe (Figure 165). This infant had acute mastoiditis requiring myringotomy and parenteral antibiotics.

Osteomyelitis

The pathogenesis of hematogenous osteomyelitis begins in the metaphysis of the tubular long bones adjacent to the epiphyseal growth plate. This avascular environment allows invading organisms to proliferate by avoiding influx of phagocytes, the presence of serum antibody and complement, interaction with tissue macrophages and other host defense mechanisms. The proliferation of organisms, release of organism-related enzymes and by-products, and the fixed volume environment contribute to the progressive bone necrosis.

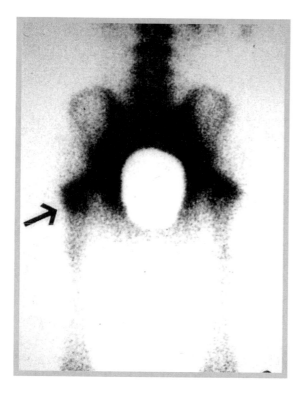

Figure 166

Signs, symptoms and pathological progression vary with the age of the patient.

The technetium-99 scan in Figure 166 of a child with osteomyelitis shows increased uptake in the right femur. Surgical drainage of the area produced 22 ml of gross pus. Gram staining of the material revealed Gram-positive cocci in clusters, and culture grew *Staphylococcus aureus*.

Bone changes on plain radiographs are not usually apparent until 7–14 days into the illness, as was the case in the infant with osteomyelitis of the proximal humerus (Figure 167) caused by group B streptococcus.

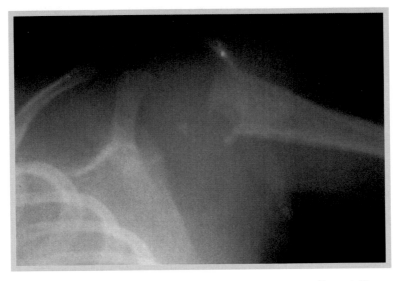

Figure 167

Septic arthritis

The diagnosis of septic arthritis is made earlier than in osteomyelitis due to the onset of constitutional symptoms within the first few days of infection. Patients almost always have fever, focal findings in the joint (swelling, tenderness, heat, limitation of motion) and placement of the joint in a neutral non-stressed position.

In infants, septic arthritis of the hip may have no focal findings except for positioning. Infants assume a position with the involved leg abducted, slightly flexed and externally rotated. Pain or resistance to motion should be evaluated for a possible septic hip. There is often an associated dislocation. An obvious portal of entry in septic arthritis is unusual.

A child had fever up to 39.5°C and a painful, tender swollen left elbow for 24 h. Needle aspiration of the joint yielded 2 ml of straw-colored fluid. Gram staining of the fluid revealed Gram-negative bacilli and culture grew *Haemophilus influenzae* type b.

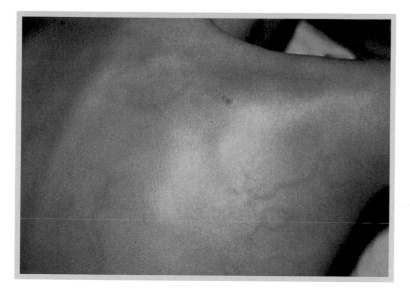

Figure 168

Other infectious diseases

Rheumatic fever

There is no laboratory test or pathognomonic clinical finding to diagnose rheumatic fever. For this reason, major and minor manifestations, described by T. Duckett Jones in 1944, are used to document the disease. Two major criteria, or one major and two minor criteria, plus supporting evidence of previous group A β-hemolytic streptococcal infection are diagnostic.

The five major criteria are carditis, migratory polyarthritis, Sydenham's chorea, erythema marginatum (Figure 168) and subcutaneous nodules (Figure 169). The minor criteria are fever, arthralgia, previous rheumatic fever or rheumatic heart disease, elevated erythrocyte sedimentation rate, positive C-reactive protein and a prolonged PR interval on electrocardiography.

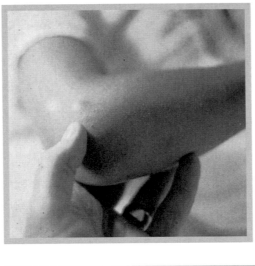

Figure 169

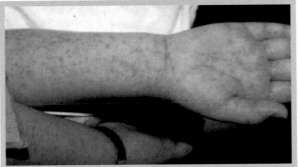

Figure 170

Ehrlichiosis

Human ehrlichiosis is a tick-borne zoonosis caused by the rickettsial organism *Ehrlichia chaffeensis*. This acute, febrile illness is clinically similar to Rocky Mountain spotted fever except that fewer than half of the patients have a rash. When present, the rash may vary from erythematous-macular to petechial (Figure 170). Other signs and symptoms, in order of frequency, are fever (95–99%), malaise (80–85%) and headache (78–84%).

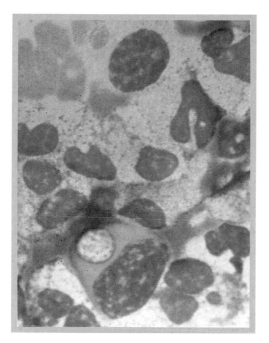

Figure 171

Although diagnosis is usually made based serologically on a four-fold or greater rise in indirect immunofluorescent titers, morulae or mulberry-like clusters of organisms may be seen in mononuclear cells in buffy-coat peripheral blood smears (Figure 171). Leukopenia and thrombocytopenia are the most consistent general laboratory abnormalities.

Rocky Mountain spotted fever

This is the most common rickettsial infection in the USA, and is caused by *Rickettsia rickettsii* and transmitted by the wood tick *Dermacentor andersoni*, the dog tick *D. variabilis* and the Lone Star tick or *Amblyomma americanum*. Organisms replicate within the endothelial lining and smooth muscle cells of blood vessels to produce a generalized vasculitis associated with a centrifugal petechial rash and fever. Hyponatremia and thrombocytopenia are frequent laboratory

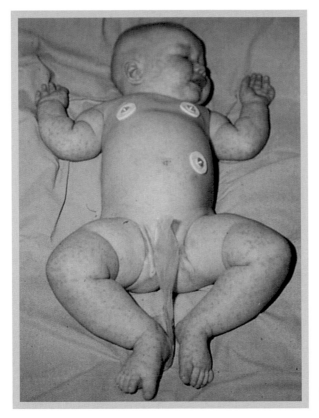

Figure 172

features. The centrifugal distribution of the rash is evident in the child with Rocky Mountain spotted fever shown in Figure 172.

A child in Virginia (Figure 173) developed fever up to 105°F for 7 days, accompanied by a maculopapular exanthem for 6 days with chills, headache, photophobia and a sore throat. Oral penicillin for 4 days was ineffective. Examination was normal except for an acutely ill, lethargic child with a generalized rash and bilateral postauricular adenopathy. Purpura and a few petechiae developed rapidly on the trunk, feet and palms. Splenomegaly was also present.

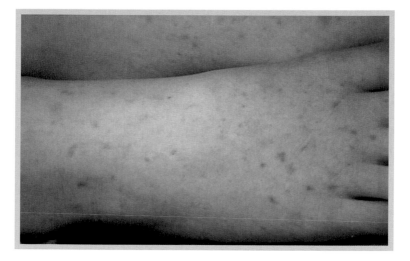

Figure 173

The Weil–Felix reaction was positive at a dilution of 1:160 for both OX-2 and OX-19 (strains of *Proteus vulgaris*), and a specific titer for Rocky Mountain spotted fever was positive at 1 : 8. Chloramphenicol was effective, with complete recovery in 6 days.

Parasitic infections

Most parasitic diseases are now well controlled in developed countries. Only pinworm (enterobiasis) and giardiasis occur frequently in pediatric practice in the USA; cases of ascariasis, amebiasis, strongyloidiasis, toxocariasis, hookworm and whipworm (trichuriasis) are only occasionally seen.

Pinworm is usually suspected in children with perianal pruritus or, rarely, vulvular pruritus. Diagnosis is confirmed by identification of *Enterobius vermicularis* eggs on clear adhesive tape (Figure 174) applied to the perianal skin when the patient first awakens in the morning. Adult nematodes, which measure 2–13 mm, may also be seen in the perianal region after the child has been asleep for a few hours.

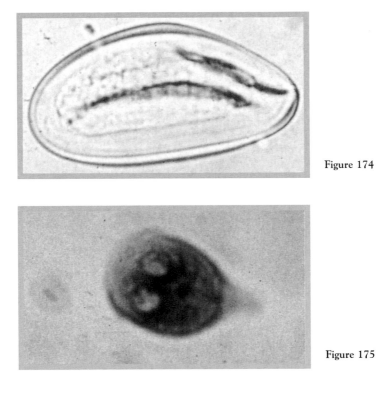

Figure 174

Figure 175

Giardia lamblia is a flagellate protozoan that produces chronic watery diarrhea accompanied by abdominal pain. Trophozoites can be identified in fresh stool specimens (Figure 175) or aspirated duodenal contents.

Ascaris lumbricoides infestation is generally asymptomatic, although non-specific gastrointestinal symptoms, transient pneumonitis (Loeffler's syndrome) and intestinal obstruction are well described. Passage of adult nematodes, which measure 15–35 mm (Figure 176), or the presence of ova in stools (Figure 177) confirms infection. The female adult worm is larger than the male (Figure 176, left) and the male has a curved tail (Figure 176, right).

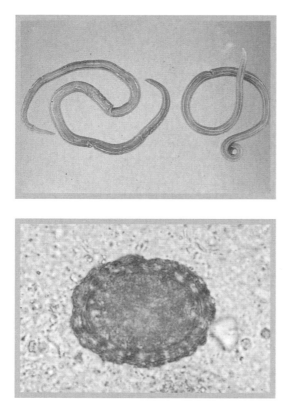

Figure 176

Figure 177

Leishmaniasis

Cutaneous leishmaniasis, a zoonotic infection, is caused by multiple species of the protozoan genus *Leishmania*. Subsequent to inoculation of parasites by the bite of an infected sandfly, local proliferation results in an erythematous macule or nodule that forms a shallow ulcer with raised borders.

Spontaneous resolution of lesions may take from weeks to years and usually results in residual scarring. The definitive diagnosis is established by microscopic identification of intracellular leishmanial

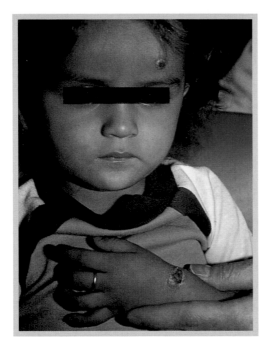

Figure 178

organisms in Giemsa-stained smears or histological sections of infected tissue.

This boy with cutaneous leishmaniasis had granulomatous ulcerations on the forehead and wrist that persisted and enlarged over a period of a month (Figure 178). He also had an enlarged epitrochlear node. The child had lived in Panama for 18 months and had been bitten by sandflies on numerous occasions.

Tissue aspiration of a granuloma revealed intracellular leishmanial organisms (amastigotes) on a Giesma-stained smear (Figure 179). Culture revealed promastigotes, clearly seen by EM. *Leishmania mexicana* was identified serologically by enzyme-linked immuno-sorbent assay (ELISA). Treatment with parenteral pentavalent antimony for 4 weeks was effective.

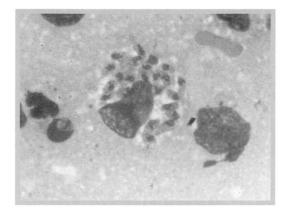

Figure 179

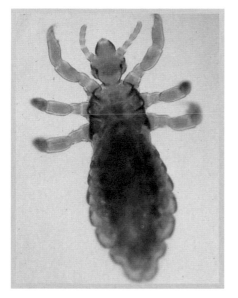

Figure 180

Pediculosis

Lice infestation in humans may involve the head, where it is caused by *Pediculus humanis capitis* (Figure 180), the body (*P. humanus corporis*), or pubic hair (*Phthirus pubis*). Transmission may be direct

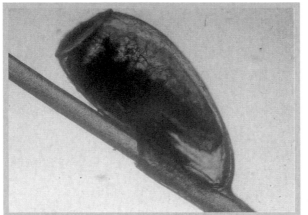

Figure 181

from contact with infected individuals or indirect (combs, brushes, etc).

The eggs (nits) are attached to hair shafts (Figure 181), and mature and hatch within 6–10 days, leaving 'empty nits' which are not infectious. Therefore, following treatment with an appropriate pediculicide, removal of nits is unnecessary and may sometimes even be painful.

Scabies

This highly contagious, intensely pruritic dermatosis is caused by the mite *Sarcoptes scabei* var. *hominis*, a parasite which lives out its entire life cycle in the stratum corneum of human skin, on which it feeds. Although pruritus may be generalized, it is most intense on the hands, wrist, axilla, waist, ankles and feet, where excoriations and burrows are most often seen (Figures 182 and 183). These are the only visible signs of the disease.

The female mite may be seen when curetted burrows or scrapings from the webbing between fingers are examined under the microscope in

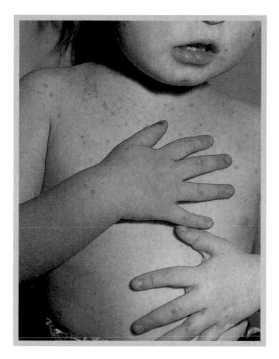

Figure 182

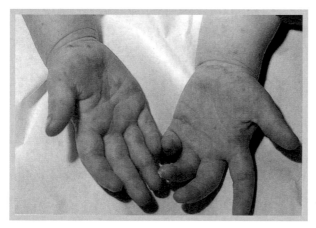

Figure 183

159

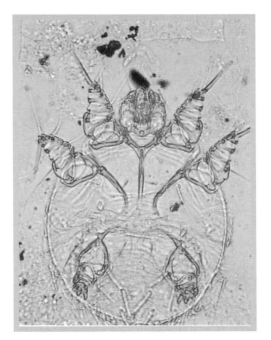

Figure 184

potassium hydroxide wet-mount preparations (Figure 184). In young infants, scabies lesions may be generalized and florid with papular, vesicular and pustular eruptions.

Pneumocystis carinii

Pulmonary infection with this fungus is closely associated with immunodeficiency, particularly in children with leukemia undergoing immunosuppressive chemotherapy and in those with AIDS caused by HIV. Disease is subacute in onset, with tachypnea, acrocyanosis and cough being the predominant signs. Crackles are often subtle and unimpressive.

Chest radiography shows diffuse bilateral alveolar and interstitial disease (Figure 185). Etiological diagnosis is made by demonstration of organisms in material from bronchoalveolar lavage, endotracheal

160

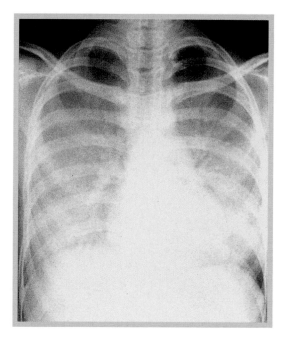

Figure 185

aspiration or open lung biopsy, using methenamine silver nitrate (Figure 186) or toluidine blue O stains.

Pseudomembranous and membranous colitis

Pseudomembranous colitis, an inflammation of the colon strongly associated with antibiotic use, is caused by *Clostridium difficile* and its toxins (A and B). Although all antibiotics have been implicated, most cases in children have been associated with ampicillin or amoxicillin. Neither the route, dosage nor duration of treatment with the antibiotic is related to development of pseudomembranous colitis.

The onset of diarrhea is sudden and patients may experience 10–20 stools/day, although children tend to have less severe diarrhea. Abdominal pain and tenderness may be present and may mimic an acute abdomen.

161

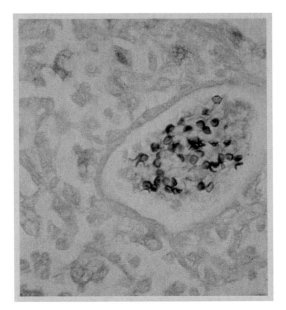

Figure 186

The treatment of pseudomembranous colitis includes fluids, supportive care and discontinuation of the offending antibiotic. Approximately 25% of patients with persistent colitis require oral antimicrobial therapy. In general, metronidazole is preferable to vancomycin. The rate of relapses is 10–20%.

Peritonitis following persistent diarrhea was seen in a premature infant who had been treated with cephalothin. There was sudden abdominal distension followed by shock and death within several hours. Autopsy revealed pseudomembranous colitis.

In contrast, a full-term infant developed severe diarrhea following removal of a meconium plug on day 2 of life. No antibiotics were given. At autopsy, extensive bronchopneumonia, peritonitis and membranous colitis were found. *Staphylococcus aureus* was cultured

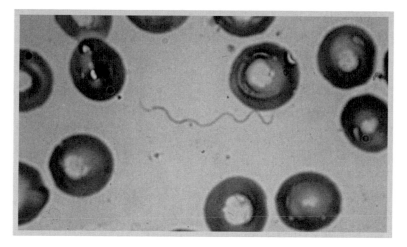

Figure 187

from the lungs and peritoneal fluid. Cystic fibrosis is the most likely cause of the infant's demise.

Relapsing fever

Spirochetes of the genus *Borrelia* produce an arthropod-borne infection characterized by recurrent high fever, chills and myalgia. Cerebrospinal pleocytosis occurs in more than 10% of cases. Disseminated disease may present with myocarditis, hepatic failure, cerebral edema or hemorrhage. Relapsing fever is more prevalent in the western parts of the USA, where disease is transmitted by soft-bodied ticks of the genus *Ornithodoros*. Louse-borne disease is endemic in east and central Africa, and in the Andes in South America.

Diagnosis is usually made by identifying the corkscrew-shaped organisms on a Wright-stained peripheral blood smear (Figure 187). Serial blood smears should be obtained during febrile episodes for maximum yield. Acridine orange-staining simplifies the screening of blood smears and is more sensitive than the traditional Wright's or Giemsa stains.

163

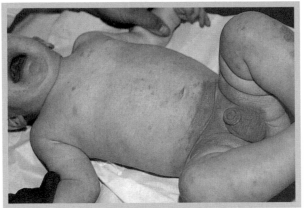

Figure 188

The immunocompromised host

Acquired immunodeficiency syndrome (AIDS)

There are a variety of initial and later clinical manifestations of HIV infection in children. Perhaps the most common manifestation is candidiasis (Figure 188), which is generally slow to resolve despite appropriate antifungal therapy. Failure to thrive with developmental delay is the second most common feature, as seen in a 10-month-old infant, who weighed 6.1 kg and was unable to sit without support. Other early findings include generalized lymphadenopathy, hepatosplenomegaly, recurrent diarrhea, *Pneumocystis carinii* pneumonia and invasive bacterial infections.

A unique early feature is parotitis (Figure 189), which tends to be recurrent but relatively painless. HIV has been isolated from biopsies of the parotid gland in these patients, suggesting that localized viral replication with accompanying cellular infiltration is the cause of enlargement.

Bacillary angiomatosis and related visceral infections are caused by *Bartonella henselae* (also the etiology of cat-scratch disease), *B. quintana*, or a related organism. Disease occurs in the immuno-

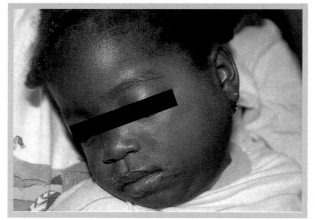

Figure 189

compromised as well as occasionally in immunocompetent patients. *Bartonella* infection of the skin, liver and spleen has been recently reported in children and adults undergoing chemotherapy for cancer. The etiology is established by positive serological tests (such as an indirect fluorescent antibody (IRA) assay), presence of silvered bacilli on Warthin–Starry staining of biopsied tissue (skin, spleen, lung nodule, bone marrow) and/or positive polymerase chain reaction for *B. quintana* or *B. henselae*.

A young AIDS patient presented with multiple generalized pink and red cutaneous angiomas measuring 3–5 mm in diameter. A larger 9-mm nodule had been noted on a finger. Biopsy of a skin lesion revealed proliferating capillaries containing large cuboidal endothelial cells with abundant cytoplasm, a characteristic feature of bacillary angiomatosis.

Chronic granulomatous disease

The majority of patients with the classical X-linked form of CGD present before the second year of life with recurrent skin infections and suppurative adenitis. Pneumonia and osteomyelitis are also common. The neutrophils of these patients are able to ingest bacteria

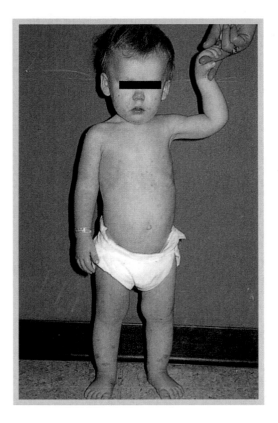

Figure 190

normally, but cannot kill catalase-producing organisms such as staphylococci, *Escherichia coli*, *Serratia marcescens*, and *Salmonella* and *Candida* species. Repeated skin infections in a child with chronic granulomatous disease healed slowly, producing multiple scars (Figure 190). His brother had died because of staphylococcal pneumonia.

Chronic mucocutaneous candidiasis

Inherited defects of T-cell and mononuclear phagocyte function produce a syndrome of persistent candidal infection of the mouth (Figure 191), scalp (Figure 192), skin (Figure 193) and nails, associ-

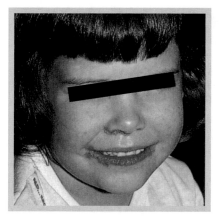

Figure 191

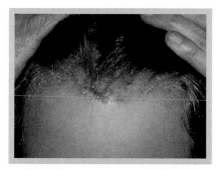

Figure 192

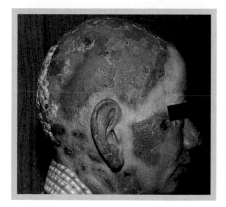

Figure 193

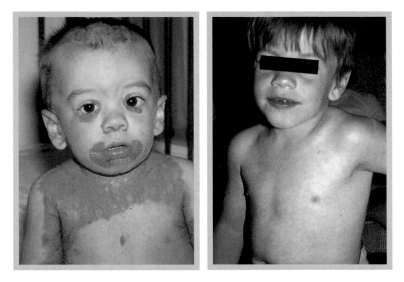

Figure 194   Figure 195

ated with endocrinopathies. Hypothyroidism and hypoparathyroidism are most commonly seen, but pancreatic and adrenal gland deficiencies have also been described. Endocrine gland dysfunction occurs months to years after candidiasis is apparent and may cause death if not recognized.

Newer antifungal agents such as ketoconazole or fluconazole are able to control mucocutaneous infection, as seen pre- and post-treatment (Figures 194 and 195) in a child with chronic mucocutaneous candidiasis.

Ecthyma gangrenosum

This is a rare but unique skin manifestation of *Pseudomonas* bacteremia, characterized by pustules or areas of cellulitis produced by septic emboli. Lesions are blackened as a consequence of hemorrhage (Figure 196) and rapidly evolve into deep ulcers with necrotic centers.

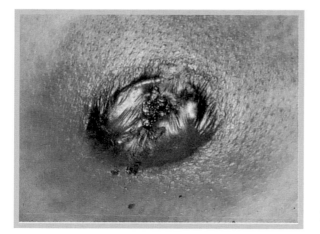

Figure 196

Patients are severely ill with predisposing factors for *Pseudomonas* infection, such as neutropenia or following placement of central intravenous catheters. Most patients are oncology patients receiving immunosuppressive chemotherapy.

Hyperimmunoglobulinemia E syndrome

The combination of recurrent staphylococcal abscesses involving the skin, lungs, joints and bones associated with serum IgE levels > 1000 IU/ml, eosinophilia and atypical atopic eczema has been attributed to an imbalance of TH-1 and TH-2 lymphocytes and is referred to as hyper IgE or Job's syndrome. The teenager in Figure 197 had deep subcutaneous abscesses caused by *Staphylococcus aureus*, a serum IgE concentration of 13 000 IU/ml and chronic eczema. His skin and lung infections began at 7 years of age. He also had a chemotactic defect of both neutrophils and monocytes.

Nocardiosis

Although all children can develop localized cutaneous or lymphocutaneous disease caused by *Nocardia* species, an invasive infection is seen in immunocompromised patients, particularly those with chronic

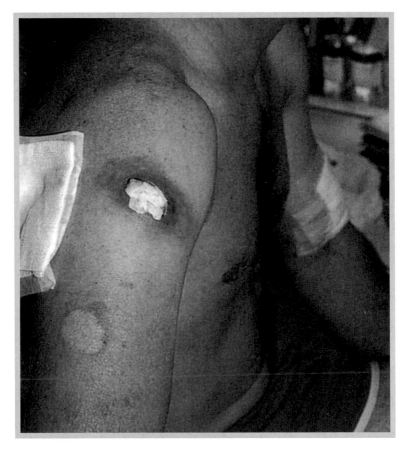

Figure 197

granulomatous disease. Infection characteristically begins in the lung with subsequent dissemination.

This boy with chronic granulomatous disease had slowly progressive pneumonia with fever lasting 1 month, after which pustular lesions appeared on his lip and face (Figure 198). Aspiration of the lip lesion

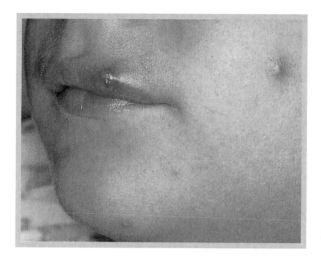

Figure 198

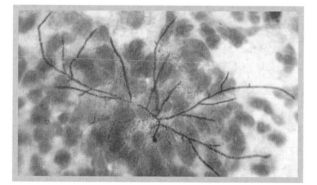

Figure 199

revealed beaded, branched, weakly Gram-positive rods in a classical asteroid configuration (Figure 199).

Noma

Also known as gangrenous stomatitis, noma is a consequence of severe malnutrition leading to tissue breakdown in the oral cavity (Figure 200) and overgrowth of *Borrelia* species or other

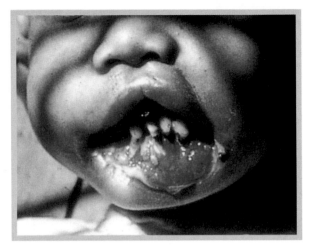

Figure 200

fusospirochetal bacteria. This infection is only seen in developing countries where kwashiorkor and marasmus are common. Initial lesions appear as small mucous membrane ulcers that rapidly extend to the skin outside of the mouth. Treatment must include nutritional support as well as high-dose penicillin and surgical debridement.

Severe combined immunodeficiency

The congenital absence of both T- and B-lymphocytes presents early in infancy with recurrent or unusual infection. Early diagnosis of this profound immune deficiency is critical, as bone marrow transplantation or enzyme replacement therapy must be provided to offer any chance of survival.

An infant, who was below the fifth centile in height and weight, had two episodes of pneumonia during the first 7 months of life. He also had an unusual chronic skin infection of his upper lip (Figure 201) that was thought to be secondary to a runny nose. Chest X-ray revealed a narrow mediastinal waist indicative of an absent thymus (Figure 202). Subsequent immunological evaluation confirmed severe combined immunodeficiency (SCID). The child underwent bone marrow transplantation with his mother as donor.

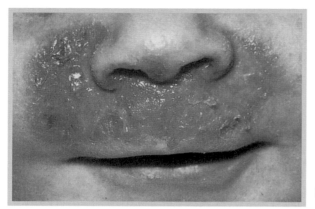

Figure 201

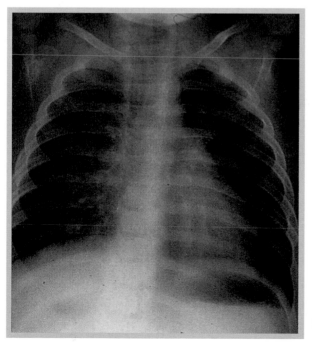

Figure 202

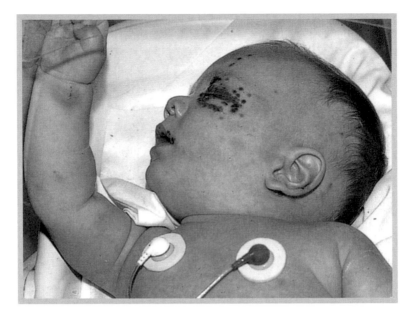

Figure 203

Wiskott–Aldrich syndrome

This X-linked recessive disease is characterized by atopic dermatitis, thrombocytopenic purpura and an increased susceptibility to infection. The initial presentation may be prolonged bleeding after circumcision secondary to the platelet defect, or recurrent or unusual infections later in life.

The patient in Figure 203 initially presented with ocular and periorbital herpes simplex infection, at which time thrombocytopenia was an incidental finding. By 18 months, he had extensive eczema (Figure 204) and, at age 3 years, severe chickenpox (Figure 205), which disseminated to the lungs and liver.

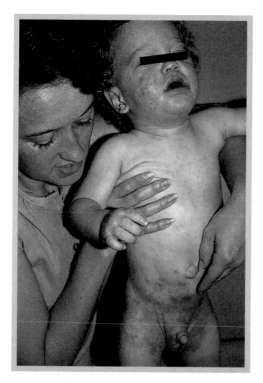

Figure 204

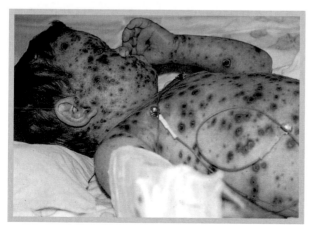

Figure 205

175

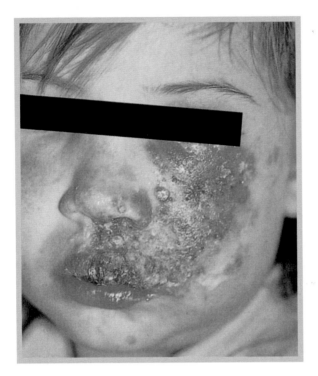

Figure 206

Zoster

Children who are immunosuppressed have an increased risk for reactivation of varicella–zoster virus (zoster or shingles). Furthermore, in those children who have malignant disorders, infection is more likely to disseminate.

The young child with leukemia in Figure 206 developed ophthalmic zoster, which was treated with intravenous acyclovir to control infection. Note that when the ophthalmic branch of the trigeminal nerve is involved, vesicles appear on the tip of the nose. In contrast, this vesicular eruption with herpes simplex (see Figure 203) does not involve the tip of the nose.

Index